WHAT I KNOW

(and the Press Isn't Telling)

The Truth Behind the Death of Donda West

by

Jan R. Adams, M.D.

ISBN: 978-0-9777778-3-9

Printed in the United States of America.

For Gwendolyn, Delia,
Kashton, Maya, Benjamin,
Alan, Bill, Griff, Nazz, Noel, N'Gai, and Wynn,
and Jonathan Edward

TABLE OF CONTENTS

ACKNOWLEDGMENTS

I would like to thank the California Medical Board, the California Department of Health Services, and the Office of the Attorney General of the State of California, my patients, nurses, plastic surgeons, and lawyers everywhere. A special thanks to Sue at Sue's Secretarial: Thank you for helping my thoughts get to paper.

PREFACE

THE TIME HAS COME TO SIMPLY TELL THE TRUTH. NOT MY TRUTH, but the facts, so that you can arrive at your own truth. You make up your own mind. Unfortunately, the truth is almost always painful or, at the very least, uncomfortable, especially to those who wish to ignore it. So long as a person doesn't know, he is free to believe what he wants.

I do not care what conclusion you choose—that is your business. I require no approval from outside myself, and I will not be owned by anyone except me. I seek only to be genuine, and I strive only to be sincere.

Jan R. Adams, M.D.

INTRODUCTION

When I pick up a new book, the first question I ask myself is: "Why should I read this?" What does it offer for me? My hope is that the author answers that question in the introduction so that I don't waste time with something that, ultimately, does not serve me. An introduction should provide the reader with a beginning knowledge or experience so that he can make an educated decision to read further.

As a physician, I am not afforded the same protections as other citizens when my reputation is challenged. Both Federal and State confidentiality laws prevent me from a public airing of details, but allows clients and the media to make virtually any statement they want regardless of its validity. And so, even before I am afforded the opportunity to respond, the tone has been set.

Regardless of the facts, I am now placed in a position where I have to defend statements made by others. Legal minds argue that those rules are in place to insure that patients feel comfortable and secure in telling the truth. My question is simply this: Why would you lie to the doctor anyway? It certainly could never serve your best interests. For that matter, why lie to anyone? The truth, as is often said, will set you free.

On the 10th of November 2007, a patient (and friend) of mine died in the post-operative period. A media circus ensued and the importance of that person to me, her family, and friends got lost in the parade of opportunists who crawled from under every conceivable rock to tell their story. None of these people were sharing the whole truth, but only portions that would serve to elevate their position. My immediate inclination was to ignore, and then to ridicule, the press, but in fact they were just as much a victim as anyone else. (That is of course, some of them. Some were willing participants in a scheme to misrepresent the facts.)

My posture in these matters is to look at things philosophically. The press, much like you and I, have been taught what to think instead of how to think. Our educational system was built to protect our way of life by developing memories in children, not abilities. What we should be teaching, however, is wisdom; and wisdom is knowledge applied. When you give someone wisdom, you do not tell them what to do or what is true, but rather how to get to their own truth. With that, and knowing the facts, I watched as the press ignored obvious truths in an attempt to persuade readers that their take was, in fact, the correct take. The press wasn't even close.

Let me say this. I take responsibility for my life and the results I get. I will not make excuses. I believe my own choices have created this opportunity for me to know who I am and to create who I wish to be. Ultimately, I thank the press for this opportunity. Know this—I will not base my sense of worthiness on the past but rather on the future. The future is clearly where my life is, not the past, and the future is clearly where my truth is. That having been said let me tell you something that you don't know.

What is Physician-Patient Privilege?

THE "PHYSICIAN-PATIENT PRIVILEGE" generally dictates that confidential communications between patient and physicians in the course of a professional relationship are privileged, and hence non-disclosable. (Evidence Code §994.) The privilege encompasses "confidential communication between patient and physician," which is defined as information transmitted between a patient and his or her physician "in the course of that relationship and in confidence by a means which, so far as the patient is aware, discloses the information to no third persons other than those who are present to further the interest of the patient in the consultation or those to whom disclosure is reasonably necessary for the transmission of the information or the accomplishment of the purpose for which the physician is consulted." The privilege covers information obtained by an examination of the patient, a diagnosis made, and the advice given by a physician in the course of that relationship. (Evidence Code §992.) The privilege applies regardless of where the patient is treated and regardless of whether the patient can communicate. (*Hale v. Superior Court (DeFelice)* (1994) 28 Cal. App.4th 1421, 34 Cal.Rptr.2d 279.)

1

"Dr. Donda West's death was not the result of an anesthesia or surgery mishap." That was the Los Angeles County Coroner speaking, and he could not have been any clearer than that. For me as a surgeon, the media circus leading up to that statement was, if not my worst, certainly in the top five of nightmares come true. A patient not under my direct care had died about 28 hours after surgery. It could have been worse from my perspective—she could have died on the operating room table, in the recovery room, or within the first 24 hours post-operatively, but she didn't. She died in the early stages of the late post-operative period, and that in itself suggested potential causes. Oddly enough, Dr. West had been abandoned early that morning by her nephew, Mr. Steven Scoggins, an experienced nurse with an advanced degree in public health to whom she had been discharged about 12 hours earlier. I say that not to condemn Mr. Scoggins; I say that merely as an observation because it will be pertinent as we follow the decedent's course as described by the coroner. (I will not comment on confidential conversations between me and Donda West, but I will comment on inaccuracies and false statements made in a public record.)

County of Los Angeles, Department of Coroner
Investigator's Narrative

Case Number: 2007-08227 Decedent: WEST, DONDA C

Information Sources:

1. Medical record #5019747, Centinela Freeman Regional Medical Center, Marina Campus. 4650 Lincoln Boulevard, Marina Del Rey, CA. 90292, 310-823-8911
2.
3.

Investigation:

On 11-12-2007 at 0746 hours E. Alonzo of Centinela Freeman Regional Medical Center reported this death to Lieutenant C. MacWillie of the Coroner's Office. The death occurred at a hospital facility and the decedent was transported to the FSC on 11-12-2007 at 0935 hours by Forensic Attendant A. Scott. Supervisor MacWillie assigned this case to me on 11-12-2007 at approximately 0900 hours.

Location:

Injury: surgical center- 11819 Wilshire Boulevard, Suite 215, Los Angeles, CA, 90025

Death: hospital- 4650 Lincoln Boulevard, Marina Del Rey, CA, 90292

Informant/Witness Statements:

Medical records were received with the decedent's incoming paperwork. The paramedic runsheet that was received was poorly copied and illegible, but it appears that when Los Angeles City Fire Department RA 63 responded to the home the decedent was in an asystolic cardiac arrest. The decedent was still in cardiac arrest when she presented to the emergency room at 2020 hours. At the time of her arrival she had been intubated and ACLS medications, including Narcan, had been administered in the field. The paramedic reported that coffee ground emesis was present to the decedent's nose. When the physician confirmed the endotracheal tube placement breath sounds were greater on the right side of the chest. The endotracheal tube was pulled back and breath sounds were then equal. Additional ACLS medications were administered, but the decedent remained asystolic throughout the resuscitative efforts. Dr. Mickey Kolodny pronounced death at 2029 hours. It was reported that the decedent had been discovered unresponsive while lying supine in bed. She had recently undergone cosmetic surgery to her breasts and abdomen. The decedent had been prescribed Keflex and Vicodin. Dr. Kolodny discussed the death with the surgeon, Dr. Jan Adams, who stated that the death should be referred to the Coroner's Office.

On the evening of 11-12-2007 I spoke with Stephen Scoggins by telephone. Mr. Scoggins is an experienced nurse and has an advanced degree in Public Health. He informed me that the decedent went for cosmetic surgery at a surgery center on 11-09-2007. The surgery started at approximately 1230 hours and at 1800 hours the decedent was in the recovery room. Mr. Scoggins received a telephone call from the decedent's friend who was concerned that she was not waking up soon enough so he responded to the surgery center. At the time of his arrival the decedent was groggy, but was oriented to person, place and time. Ms. West had arranged for caregivers to stay with her during the night and the group returned to the decedent's home. Mr. Scoggins also stayed at the home and stated that the decedent ambulated during the night to prevent a deep vein thrombosis from forming. She was in pain and was medicated with Vicodin. In the morning the decedent stated that she felt better and was able to ambulate without assistance. Mr. Scoggins stated that the decedent appeared to be doing well so he left for the day with the intention to return and spend the night with his aunt. The decedent was left with caregivers Diana and Nubia who had been referred by Dr. Adams in addition to her friend, Glenda. At the time Mr. Scoggins left he stated that the decedent did not appear to be diaphoretic and had no symptoms of peritonitis or bleeding. Mr. Scoggins stated that the

Figure 1

County of Los Angeles, Department of Coroner
Investigator's Narrative

Case Number: 2007-08227 Decedent: WEST, DONDA C.

decedent had no known cardiac problems or peptic ulcer disease. There is no history of substance abuse.

On the evening of 11-12-2007 I spoke with the decedent's long-time friend, Glenda Lee, by telephone. She informed me that the decedent had consulted with four doctors before selecting Dr Adams to perform a breast augmentation, "tummy tuck" and liposuction of her lower back. The decedent had a history of thyroid problems and took Synthroid. At one time she had been diagnosed with hypertension, but said that it had gone away; she was not taking anti-hypertensive medication The decedent was also a border-line diabetic She had seen physicians in the past at UCLA Medical Center in Westwood and Cedars-Sinai Medical Center Two weeks before the surgery the decedent had experienced some leg pain, but did not see a doctor and the cause was unknown Ms. Lee reported that heart problems run in the family and the decedent's sister died two years ago of a "heart attack." Her brother has a history of hypertension. It is unknown whether Ms. West had undergone any specialized tests prior to her surgery. Ms. Lee stated that she had arrived at the decedent's home on 11-10-2007 at 1600 hours. The two caregivers had gotten her out of bed and a few blood spots were seen on the abdominal dressing. The decedent had been ambulated every two hours and she was receiving Vicodin for her pain. At the time of Ms. Lee's arrival the decedent stated that her throat was hurting and her chest was hurting. The chest discomfort was felt to be the result of the breast augmentation and the tight bandages. The decedent felt warm to touch and at 1630 hours she ate some chicken soup, crackers, water and pineapple juice before her medications were given. The decedent was described as having "a lot of pain." Ms. Lee stated that she sat with her friend and rubbed her neck. She noticed that the decedent was "breathing heavy." At 1700 hours Ms. West went to bed and at that time she said that her chest was tight and her throat was sore. The decedent again got out of bed, but was not described as being anxious or confused. When she went back to bed pillows were beneath her legs and a single pillow was beneath her head. The decedent was able to tolerate lying flat. Ms. Lee went to the kitchen for a short while and when she returned the decedent had "black stuff on her face" and was cold and clammy. When her pulse was noted to be absent 911 was called. As rescue breaths were given more "blood" drained from the decedent's nose.

Scene Description:

The scene was not visited by coroner personnel.

Evidence:

No physical or medical evidence was collected for this report

Body Examination:

The decedent was seen lying on a tray inside the FSC service floor She is an adult female approximately 65-inches in length and weighs approximately 188 pounds. She has brown braided hair brown eyes and natural teeth. An endotracheal tube was secured in her mouth and electrocardiogram patches and defibrillator pads were noted to her torso The decedent had steri-striped incisions to her breasts and lower abdomen Jackson-Pratt drains were intact to both anterior hip areas and the umbilicus had sutures. Viewing the decedent's back was deferred to the pathologist due to the instability of the tray

Identification:

The decedent was identified by her nephew, Stephen Scoggins, while at the hospital

Figure 1 (continued)

Mr. Scoggins reported to the coroner that he "received a telephone call on the day of surgery" from the decedent's friend "who was concerned that she was not waking up soon enough after surgery, so he responded to the Surgery Center". He may in fact have received a call, but not for those reasons. Dr. West was awake. We were waiting for the nurse, Mr. Scoggins, to arrive so that the patient could be discharged to the person who was responsible for her post-op care. I was told by her sister and my staff that Mr. Scoggins was getting equipment and preparing Dr. West's bedroom for her recovery. That supposedly was why he was late picking her up. It is our policy to discharge patients to their caregivers so that post-operative orders can be given directly to those people responsible for the patient's post-operative care.

My problem with Mr. Scoggins' statement is that it is a bit too casual. Stephan Scoggins is not a concerned bystander in this matter. He is very much an active participant. It was Mr. Scoggins who convinced his aunt that he would take care of her post-operatively and therefore did not need an aftercare facility; it was Mr. Scoggins who assured her that surgery would be the right thing to do because he would be with her throughout the process (understand Donda West had scheduled and cancelled surgery, many times with many doctors); and it was Mr. Scoggins who convinced his aunt to sign an advanced directive giving him power of attorney over her affairs.

Mr. Scoggins arrived around 7 p.m. dressed in a short white lab coat. He informed me that he was Dr. Scoggins and that he would be taking care of his aunt. He apologized that his family was "a little crazy", and offered that he and Donda were, in fact, "the backbone of that family". He also requested other medications for her at the time. I declined to prescribe them, informing him that I do not prescribe a medicine with side effects to combat the side effects of another medicine. I did offer, however, that I would check-up on them later. If at that time she needed other medications I would make the arrangements. With that, Donda West, his aunt, was discharged to his care.

Further along in the coroner's report, it is reported by Mr. Scoggins that "the decedent was left with caregivers, Diana and Nubia, who had been referred by Dr. Adams." But that could not be further from the truth. First of all, neither of these people had been referred to Ms. West as caregivers. I had referred Ms. West to Nirvana, an after-care facility, but she opted to be taken care of by Mr. Scoggins, a registered nurse with an advanced degree, but more importantly, her nephew.

Nubia was Dr. West's personal assistant (and surely Mr. Scoggins knew that). Diana was a former patient of ours with whom Dr. West had formed a friendship (and surely Mr. Scoggins knew this also).

As is our policy, if a prospective patient wishes to speak with former patients who have had similar procedures, we try to arrange it so that they can get together. The patient can then get an informed perspective on how other people were treated by us. Diana was not the only previous patient of ours with whom Dr. West had communicated. Nonetheless, they had hit it off and Diana had apparently committed to spending time with Ms. West in her immediate post-operative period. The point is that neither individual was referred by our office as caregivers.(By the way, I corrected this statement with Ms. Denice Bertone RN, the coroner's investigator, at the suggestion of Ms Robin Hollis, an investigator for the Medical Board of California. Ms. Bertone's reply: "I knew he wasn't being truthful. Why would a doctor refer as caregivers two people who aren't even LPN's? People lie to us all the time, but I can recheck my notes. I pretty sure that's what he said … My job is to take the statement as people give it.")

Even more alarming, Mr. Scoggins claims to have been a police officer in the state of Oklahoma and surely, a former police officer knows that lying to the coroner is a crime.

To continue with the coroner's report, Mr. Scoggins stated that "the decedent appeared to be doing well so he left for the day with the intention to return and spend the night with his aunt". (Yet prior to leaving, when Donda complained of pain, a sore throat, and chest tightness (according to a declaration by Ms. Diane Pinckney), he told her she had a pneumonia. So if you thought someone had a pneumonia, wouldn't you call her doctor. Mr. Scoggins didn't.) At the time Mr. Scoggins left, as stated in the coroner's report, "the decedent did not appear to be diaphoretic and had no symptoms of peritonitis or bleeding. Mr. Scoggins stated that the decedent had no known cardiac problems or peptic ulcer disease".

As one of my favorite people, the Rev. Dr. J. Alfred Smith, Sr. of the Allen Temple Baptist Church in Oakland, California, would say, "Let me say that again so the whole congregation and not just the choir might get it." Mr. Scoggins stated that the decedent had no known cardiac problems or peptic ulcer disease. (That is of particular importance because throughout the media frenzy reporters refer to Dr. West's heart problems.) Furthermore, it is important to point out, as also noted by the coroner's report, that the decedent's previous medical history included evaluation for an episode of left chest and arm pain on January 10, 2007 at Cedars-Sinai Medical Center. *No prior history of heart disease was noted.* The decedent indicated a previous history of elevated cholesterol, and hypothyroid disease treated with Synthroid. Chest x-ray and cardiac workup were unremarkable. *Again we have a cardiac workup done at Cedars-Sinai Medical Center that was unremarkable.*

By the way, as a courtesy, I sent a copy of the letter addressed to the coroner to the lawyers of Mr. Scoggins and the estate of Donda West informing them of the inaccuracies in the coroner's report.

JAN ADAMS MEDICAL GROUP, INC.
11819 Wilshire Blvd., Suite 214
Los Angeles, CA 90025
Telephone (310) 444-8808 Facsimile (310) 444-8809

March 7, 2008

Louis Peña, M.D.
Department of Coroner
County of Los Angeles
1104 N. Mission Road
Los Angeles, CA 90033

Dear Dr. Peña:

A Ms. Robin Hollis, an investigator with the Medical Board of California, visited my office on Wednesday, March 5, 2008, requesting records for Donda West. As a result, I reviewed the coroner's report. I noted a number of not only inaccurate but frankly false statements made by Ms. West's nephew, Stephan Scoggins, RN. In his statement Mr. Scoggins' states that he was present as a favor to his aunt and that the other people were caregivers. That statement by Nurse Scoggins is completely false. He was, in fact, the primary caregiver. I released Dr. West to Nurse Scoggins, and the other people Scoggins mentions in his statement were merely friends and/or employees of Ms. West.

Scoggins told your investigator that the decedent was left with caregivers, Diana and Nubia, who had been referred by Dr. Adams. Mr. Scoggins certainly knows that Nubia was Dr. West's personal assistant, and that Diana was a recent friend of Dr. West. Again, neither Nubia nor Diana were referred to Ms. West as caregivers. I am concerned that the grossly inaccurate and false statements made to your investigator by Mr. Scoggins were an attempt to deflect attention from his behavior. It would appear to me that an experienced nurse with an advanced degree in public health, who had offered to manage his aunt's postoperative care, would be more diligent and that he would not have abandoned her the next morning. Dr. West had designated Scoggins as her primary care giver in her Advanced Directive which she signed on the day of surgery. We had previously made arrangements for Dr. West to be cared for at Nirvana aftercare facility. However, Dr. West decided that she preferred to be under the care of nurse Scoggins and at her own home. Additionally, contrary to Scoggins' statement about the reason for the delay in Dr. West's release, in fact the delay was due to the late arrival of nurse Scoggins who had indicated that he was getting medical equipment, including a wheelchair and monitor, for Dr. West's care at home. We later learned that he had in fact not picked up any equipment for the Dr. West's recovery. Without these monitoring equipments it makes the fact that he entrusted Dr. West's care to people without medical training even more outrageous.

Figure 2

Louis Peña, M.D.
March 7, 2008
Page 2

Nurse Scoggins would like to minimize his involvement in this matter, however, he was the primary care giver, he was the person who picked up Dr. West from the Surgery center, and he was the person designated by Dr. West to be in charge of her care according to an advanced directive signed by Dr. West.

Further, Scoggins is the personal representative for the estate of Dr. West and his assertion of the estate's HIPPA privilege in order to prevent me from discussing the case is nothing more than an attempt to cover up his misconduct which is certainly not a proper purpose for asserting the privilege.

At the suggestion of Ms. Hollis, I will take a close look at the coroner's report to see if there are any other inaccuracies which should be corrected in that this file is a public record.

Please let me know how you intend to proceed with this matter.

Sincerely,

Jan R. Adams, M.D.

CC: Robin Hollis, Medical Board of California

Brentwood Surgery Center, Inc.

McPherson & Associates

Thomas Byrnes, Esq.

Figure 2 (continued)

The coroner's office, as had been my experience, was diligent in getting back to me, and confirmed receipt of my letter advising them of the inaccuracies in Mr. Scoggins' statement. Mr. Brad Rose, of Pryor Cashman LLP in New York City, the "litigation counsel to the Estate of Dr. Donda West and the surviving personal representatives of Dr. West" was not so diligent. It took my letter, a letter from my attorney, and four telephone calls to him to even get him to acknowledge receipt of the letter.

COUNTY OF LOS ANGELES

DEPARTMENT OF CORONER

1104 N. MISSION RD., LOS ANGELES, CALIFORNIA 90033

"Enriching Lives"

Anthony T. Hernandez
Director

Lakshmanan Sathyavagiswaran, M.D.
Chief Medical Examiner-Coroner

March 13, 2008

Dr. Jan R. Adams
Brentwood Surgery Center, Inc.
11819 Wilshire Blvd., Suite 214
Los Angeles, CA 90025

Dear Dr. Adams:

We received your letter from March 7, 2008 and it has been reviewed along with the Chief Medical Examiner-Coroner Dr. Lakshmanan Sathyavagiswaran and Investigator Coroner and RN Ms. Denise Bertone.

We will follow up on the concerns raised in your letter.

Sincerely,

Louis A. Pena, M.D.
Deputy Medical Examiner
Los Angeles County- Department of Coroner

Accreditations:

National Association of Medical Examiners
California Medical Association-Continuing Medical Education
Accreditation Council for Graduate Medical Education
American Society of Crime Laboratory Directors
Peace Officer Standards and Training Certified

Law and Science Serving the Community

Figure 3

In the meantime, I had forwarded another letter to Mr. Rose dated the 8th of April, 2008. I was getting frustrated with his silence because I had been more than fair and genuine with him.

JAN ADAMS MEDICAL GROUP, INC.
11819 Wilshire Blvd., Suite 214
Los Angeles, CA 90025
Telephone (310) 444-8808 Facsimile (310) 444-8809

April 8, 2008

Sent 4/8/08

Mr. Brad Rose, Esq.
Pryor Cashman LLP
410 Park Avenue, 10th Floor
New York, NY 10022

Dear Brad:

I am writing to follow up on several telephone calls I made to you to which you have not responded.

My concern is related to action taken by you and McPhearson on behalf of Dr. Scoggins in his capacity as personal representative of the estate of Donda West.

I am deeply offended by the conduct of Dr. Scoggins. Dr. West suggested that she had a great deal of respect for his professional competence. In fact she decided to entrust her after surgery care to him rather than being cared for at the recovery center which we had arranged for her. Had she gone to the recovery center, or had Scoggins performed his duties as he said he would, the outcome may have been very different. Whether his conduct rises to the level of gross negligence is an open question at this point. However, Scoggins did make misleading and some frankly false statements to the coroner and this raises serious questions as to his motives. Innocent people don't need to lie. Nonetheless, this eventually will be sorted out by the proper authorities.

My concern with respect to you and Mr. McPherson is that after Dr. Scoggins gave his statement to the coroner on 11/12/07, you took a number of actions which prevented me from defending myself from false and misleading statements made in the press by asserting the doctor patient privilege. The false statements made by Scoggins to the coroner confirm that the purpose of these efforts was to protect Dr. Scoggins and his actions from scrutiny not the privacy of Donda West. The corner's report clears me and the Surgery Center of any misconduct, but does not clearly address the role that Scoggins' conduct may have had in contributing to her death. His lies to the coroner at that time had the effect of hiding material information about his role in the events which lead up to her death.

Figure 4

Surely I have no evidence nor would I suggest that you or McPherson were aware of Scoggings' role when you took steps to protect him, but their effect on my reputation my medical practice and on Brentwood surgery center have been devastating. Basically actions that were taken on behalf of your client have destroyed my practice and destroyed Brentwood surgery center. Regardless of your involvement or knowledge of the underlying facts, the effects of your actions have been the same.

My purpose in contacting you was to discuss this new information and decide what needed to be done to be fair to everybody. My feeling is that if Scoggins would lie to the coroner's investigator about the events that led to Donda's death, he will certainly lie to the authorities with respect to what he told his attorneys and what his attorneys told him to say and do after Donda's death.

I know that given your representation of Scoggins this may raise conflict of interest issues which you and Mr. McPherson may need to resolve. If you are not the person who I should be calling, let me know who I should contact.

Sincerely,

Jan Adams, MD

Figure 4 (continued)

To my surprise, shortly after that, my attorney, Mr. Michael Payne, called to inform me that he had received a letter addressed to him from Mr. Rose. He faxed a copy to my office and after reading it, I went through the roof. I was being fair and this guy was continuing to be a prick. I immediately tried to call his office, and when he wouldn't take the call, I sat down to write him a very nasty (but professional) letter. (Which, by the way, I never sent to him.)

04/24/2008 14:13 6269748712 PAYNE PAGE 02/02

PRYOR CASHMAN LLP

New York | Los Angeles

410 Park Avenue, New York, NY 10022 Tel: 212-421-4100 Fax: 212-326-0806

www.pryorcashman.com

Brad D. Rose
Partner

Direct Tel: 212-326-0875
Direct Fax: 212-798-6369
brose@pryorcashman.com

March 25, 2008

VIA FACSIMILE & U.S. MAIL

Michael D. Payne. Esq.
Wells Fargo Bank Building
433 North Camden Drive, Ste. 400
Beverly Hills, CA 90210

Re: Dr. Jan Adams

Dear Mr. Payne:

Reference is made to your letter to me dated February 28, 2008 as well as to the March 7, 2008 letter that Dr. Adams allegedly transmitted to the Los Angeles County Coroner's Office. Reference is further made to the voice message that Dr. Adams left for me at my office on March 24, 2008. Please be advised that, in response to your request, the Estate of Donda West will not waive the physician/patient privilege. In addition, I have also been asked to caution Dr. Adams from continuing to publish false and defamatory statements concerning Dr. West's nephew, Stephan Scoggins.

Thank you for your attention to these matters.

Sincerely,

Brad D. Rose

BDR:mar

700992

Figure 5

JAN ADAMS MEDICAL GROUP, INC.
11819 Wilshire Blvd., Suite 214
Los Angeles, CA 90025
Telephone (310) 444-8808 Facsimile (310) 444-8809

April 30, 2008

Mr. Brad D. Rose, Esq.
Law Offices, Pryor Cashman LLP
410 Park Avenue
New York, NY 10022

Re: Response to Letter sent to Michael Payne, March 28, 2008

Dear Mr. Rose,

I received a facsimile copy of a letter dated March 25, 2008, addressed to my attorney Michael D. Payne, Esq. This is the second time you're made threatening remarks and now I'm done with it. I've made every attempt to discuss this matter with you as a gentleman and you have, along with your client, been dishonest, all along the way.

The fact of the matter is that I have made four attempts by phone to discuss with you the misleading and false statements made by your client, Stephan Scoggins, to the LA County Coroner. On each occasion your secretary put me on hold, and then came back to say either that you were not in, or not available, and that she would give you the message.

On the 24th of March I informed her that she had told me that a number of times before over the past few weeks and then she got testy, telling me "all she could do was give you the message." I guess she got tired of lying for you too.

Frankly, I knew that you and Stephan Scoggins would not waive the physician-patient privilege for the Estate of Donda West because both of you have things to hide.

Mr. Scoggins wants to hide that he convinced his aunt not to go to Nirvana, the aftercare facility; he wants to hide that he insisted she sign an advanced directive putting him in charge of her estate; he wants to hide that he was late picking his aunt up from the surgery center under the guise of getting her room ready for recovery, and yet got none of the equipment he said he was getting; he wants to hide that he, a nurse with an advanced degree, abandoned his aunt the next morning to go to a baby shower (a baby shower for Christ's sake); he wants to hide the fact that he left two women there with no medical

Figure 6

training whatsoever to take care of her, and then refused to answer their calls; he wants to hide that he turned his phone off so he wouldn't be bothered; he wants to hide that for 12 hours (the time he left until the time he saw her body at the hospital) he made no inquiries about his aunt; and then lastly, he wants to hide that he, as a former police officer, lied to the coroner about his involvement.

The last part is particularly disturbing because I am now sure by your posture that you knew all this before you wrote your initial letter to me on November 13, 2007. While Harvey Levin and TMZ tried to invoke themselves as the "lead dog" in this media frenzy, you knew I had not discussed Donda West with them because they had it all wrong.

For instance, when asked by Larry King "what do we know?"

Harvey said "well, first of all we know the surgery took 8 hours which already tells us something went wrong."

The surgery took 5 l/2 hours and the coroner's report confirmed that. Had he discussed it with me he would have surely gotten that right. Nonetheless, Harvey continued to share inaccuracies with Larry King demonstrating he didn't get his information from the surgeon.

Harvey Levin was getting his information from you and Scoggins. In order to hide his negligence Scoggins' (along with your help) pitch was that I was responsible for Donda's death and that you guys needed to pull out all stops to make sure I paid for it. Your game plan was not to get the Medical Board of California to revoke my license but to get the DA to prosecute me for involuntary manslaughter based on a criminal negligence theory. If I was prosecuted, Scoggins would be totally off the hook.

The problem is that your fabricated version wasn't supported by the facts of the case. I thank God every day that the LA County Coroner's Office is not only professional, thorough, and good at what they do, but that they are honest also.

But that's why you and Ed McPherson went to such lengths to shut me up. That's why you went so far as to file complaints with the Medical Board, even going so far as to implicate Kanye West himself by having him sign an "undated complaint" against Brentwood Surgery Center.

So here's what I can assure you: while I don't know him personally, Michael Gargiulo, who is a Deputy District Attorney, is very sharp and it won't take him long to figure this all out.

Figure 6 (continued)

Rather than making inappropriate threats and accusations against me, I suggest that you concentrate on how to eventually explain to your client, Kanye West, that the person most responsible for his mother's death is the person sitting in the room with you. Furthermore, that you and McPherson, through your heavy-handed tactics to shut me up while you helped the press defame me and the authorities including the Department of Health Services and the Medical Board of California disrupt business at Brentwood Surgery Center, have been protecting Scoggins all along. Explain to your client why his lawyers not only have a "conflict of interest" in representing both Stephan Scoggins and the Estate of Donda West, but that they may also be parties to "obstruction of justice" because they knew all along Scoggins was lying to the Coroner.

Now, let me be clear that I hate having to talk with you like this but make no doubt I have had enough. Don't mistake kindness for weakness.

Warm Regards

Jan R. Adams, MD

Figure 6 (continued)

The press, however, ignored the facts in the coroner's report, and the facts of the case, all of them. They were looking for someone to crucify and no amount of truth or facts were going to get in their way. But wait, I'm getting ahead of myself. To truly understand how a media circus and misinformation like this that surrounded the death of Donda West got started, you must first get a glimpse into the press and how they work.

2

"Think of the press as a process, not as a thing." (Micheal Sitrick/Allan Mayer, "Spin" 1995) The press is comprised of a group of people, each with their own beliefs, hopes, desires, and prejudices. They have, however, one thing in common: they love telling a story. A story has a beginning, middle, and an end with as much drama, and unsuspected twists and turns as possible. There are clear-cut victims and villains and the end must always bring the drama to a satisfactory conclusion. There can be no loose ends.

The majority of people involved in this process see themselves as the moral compass of society. They are drawn to journalism because they truly want to champion the right, and expose the wrong. They want to make the world better.

Journalism is also a very competitive business where one must prove himself every hour of every day. It boils down to this: did you get the story first? Did you meet that deadline? The pressure must be enormous and as with enormous pressure comes the recipe for mistakes. (I really don't have time to check the facts. I have to get the story out first.)

Journalists also want to own the story. They want to define the issue and set the tone. They want to be seen as the seasoned insider who not only gets the story first, but gets it right. They don't want the official story; they want the real story. They want the angle to the story that no other journalist can get, and that is where the problem lies. The pressure to be first; the desire to be the one who defines the issue; and the need to be recognized for that serve to create an environment where the journalist can find himself creating the story and not merely reporting the story. Ego takes over, and the "lead dog" takes the pack of journalists who follow, down the same path. We live in a nanosecond world and information can be sent around the globe in real time. The problem occurs when the lead dog gets it wrong. That is precisely what happened in the case of Donda West. The press got it wrong.

I recognize that the press must constantly feed that beast: that they have an hour of news to fill, or an article to print every day. I recognize that they have that piece to write each week regardless of what's going on in the world. If nothing newsworthy is happening that day, too bad. The six o'clock news still has to come on, and that newspaper or magazine still has to go out.

For the press, what happened in Dr. West's case was a godsend. You had the mother of a famous musical artist, you had a celebrity plastic surgeon with a television show, and unfortunately—or fortunately, depending on how you look at it—you had an untimely death.

Unfortunately, also, what you didn't have was information. That celebrity plastic surgeon is also a doctor and there are laws which prevent doctors, lawyers, and the clergy from discussing the privileged information of their clients.

Now the press hates when they have nothing to say. They simply can't tolerate a time when they can't fill that hour or place that article in a newspaper or magazine. Since they couldn't talk with the doctor or penetrate the circle of that music star, they created their own story.

They allowed the story be defined by an internet tabloid reporter named Harvey Levin. Mr. Levin called my answering service Monday evening, two days after her death. He introduced himself and his company, neither of which I had ever heard, and began to rattle off questions. I confirmed that I was indeed Ms. West's surgeon and ask that he respect the family, and that was essentially the context of our phone call. Mr. Levin, it seems, is not one to be put off and kept asking a barrage of questions. I informed him that I didn't want to be rude to him but that I wasn't going to answer specific questions about my patient. I did tell him, however, that if and when it became appropriate, and that if he was fair to the family, I would give him and his organization my first interview. I might add however, he did neither.

To my surprise, this Mr. Levin ended up on "Larry King Live" and without a story to peddle, he made one up. In transcripts of the show, Mr. Levin began by saying that he called me and then I (TRANSCRIPTS: CNN LARRY KING LIVE Aired November 13, 2007- 21:00 ET) called him back. That's not true. My service called to say that there was a man on the line saying he's calling about a patient but won't tell them who the patient is. I asked them to put him through. The operator offered that he's lying and I said I know, but we shouldn't take the chance, it really could be a patient who needs me.

Larry King asked "Harvey, What do we know?"

Harvey Levin replied, "Well, we know a lot, we know the surgery took eight (8) hours which already tells you there was a problem".

But now we have a coroner's report and not just Harvey's word: THE OPERATION TOOK FIVE AND ONE-HALF HOURS, NOT EIGHT. Harvey was wrong. Where was Harvey getting his information? He was not getting it from me the surgeon. He had misled Larry King and the rest of America by saying he had talked with me (which was true) but he was relaying information that clearly didn't come from me (which is also very true).

Harvey was using an old tabloid trick to fool the public and the rest of the media. I think it's fair to say I would have known the length of the operation and clearly would not have told him something untrue to make myself look bad. If a surgeon is going to tell you about a procedure he performed, I can guarantee his recollection of time will be shorter not longer.

Harvey went on to say "the surgery should have taken four hours".

Where did he get that? Not from me. In fact, now that we do have a coroner's report, and know what procedures she had, I challenge Harvey or anyone else to query plastic surgeons and produce five who could get that done in less than eight hours. The point is this: THE CORONER WAS RIGHT: NEITHER SURGERY NOR ANESTHESIA MISHAPS CONTRIBUTED TO DONDA WEST'S DEATH.

Harvey Levin then said, "I'm told she should have gone to a recovery center. This is a pretty big operation. She didn't. And she may not have gone because she had this condition and they may not have wanted her there because she was high risk."

Once again what on earth is Mr. Levin talking about and where is he getting his information: certainly not from me, the surgeon. He is trying to convince everybody he had this in depth conversation with me, but his information is wrong.

What is her condition? Again, Cedar Sinai Medical Center evaluated her and discharged her home with the results unremarkable. It's in the coroner's report. (Also, I can say that Dr. Aboolian, who Mr. Levin quotes, is less than genuine. If, indeed he evaluated her as he says on TV, then surely he knows what I know, and what I know is that he and Mr. Levin aren't presenting the facts. He and Mr. Levin are using Ms. West's death to promote themselves. Furthermore, Mr. Scoggins and his attorneys Brad Rose and Ed McPherson could resolve this entire issue by releasing me from the constraints of the doctor-patient privilege and allowing the facts to be presented. But they won't, and therein Mr. Levin is the story. The coroner has made his determination, along with expert pathologists from UCLA, USC, and the West family's own pathologist that *I recommended they get.* Why then Mr. Levin don't they want us to know what happen once she left the surgery center? Who or what are they hiding?)

"So he sent her home and she died" concluded Mr. Levin to Larry King.

But she wasn't just sent home Mr. Levin. Donda West was released to the care of her nephew, Dr. Stephan Scoggins, an experienced nurse with an advanced degree. (It says so in the coroner's report.) He had consented to take care of his aunt and apparently that was why she didn't go to an aftercare facility. He had prepared her room for recovery with beds, chairs, and monitors. He had had her sign power of attorney over to him. He picked her up, and, once again, he took her home.

The problem is Harvey Levin got it wrong. And what he didn't get wrong, in typical tabloid fashion; he told only half the story. This was about putting a camera on Harvey. That is what Harvey wanted. He wasn't the sophisticated insider who got it first; he was the naïve clown who got it wrong. And when it seemed the camera was going to be taken off of him, little Harvey got nasty.

He began by attacking the issue of board certification, but Harvey didn't really understand the significance of what it meant:

The American Board of Plastic Surgery certifies that the PLASTIC SURGERY PROGRAMS across the country meet certain minimum required standards by testing those individuals who have completed a certain minimum of requirements to sit for their exams.(What they are really examining is the program, not specifically the individual. This was also suggested to Amy Keith, a writer for People Magazine, by Dr. David A. Kulber, director of the Plastic Surgery Center at Cedar Sinai in Los Angeles. His quote: "{noncertification} suggests a problem in your training or education". She ignored that.)

Examination of the American Board of Plastic Surgery Inc. *Booklet on Information* dated July 1, 2007 to June 30, 2008, says this;

> "For Physicians with Medical or Osteopathic Degrees granted in the United States or Canada, and for International Medical Graduates, one of the following pathways must be taken:

I. For residents entering plastic surgery residency training in 2009 or after, a minimum of five progressive years of clinical training in general surgery sufficient to qualify for certification by ABS is required. The satisfactory completion of this requirement must be verified in writing by the general surgery program director. As previously noted, effective July 1, 2009, if completing less than full general surgery training, plastic surgery training must be completed in the same institution as the general surgery training. The Accreditation Council for Graduate Medical Education (ACGME) or the Royal College of Physicians and Surgeons in Canada (RCPSC) so you must accredit both the programs. Broad surgical training experience is required.

A total of 36 months of general surgery is required. A **minimum** of 18 months must be devoted to rotations in the essential areas of general surgery as listed in categories 1 through 12 below:

1. General Surgery
2. Alimentary Tract Surgery
3. Abdominal Surgery
4. Breast Surgery
5. Head and Neck Surgery
6. Vascular Surgery
7. Endocrine Surgery
8. Surgical Oncology
9. Trauma
10. Critical Care
11. Pediatric Surgery
12. Transplant

During the 36 months of general surgery, no more than a total of 12 months may be served in the other areas of surgical training such as:

1. Gynecology
2. Neurologic surgery
3. Ophthalmology

4. Orthopedic surgery
5. Otolaryngology
6. Urology
7. Anesthesia
8. Burns
9. Surgical pathology
10. Surgical dermatology
11. Oral and maxillofacial surgery
12. Cardiothoracic surgery

During the 36 months of general surgery, the limitations on the time spent in the specified rotations must include not more than:

- 1 month on pathology or dermatology
- 2 months on oral and maxillofacial surgery
- 3 months on a single rotation of the other subspecialties
- 6 months on the combination of plastic surgery and hand surgery

II. Alternate Prerequisite Pathways Accepted

An accredited residency training program in neurological surgery, orthopedic surgery, otolaryngology, or urology is accepted.

Prospective candidates may initiate resident training in plastic surgery following satisfactory completion of the entire course of training in the United States or Canada, as prescribed for certification by the American Board of Neurological Surgery, the American Board of Orthopaedic Surgery, the American Board of Otolaryngology, or the American Board of Urology. Prospective candidates **must** meet and comply with the most current requirements in these specialties. Satisfactory completion of training **must** be verified in writing by the training program director (see Verification of Prerequisite Training) and evidence of current admissibility to the respective ABMS specialty board's examination process in the United States must be provided.

III. For prospective candidates with an M.D. degree obtained in the United States or Canada combined with a dental degree (D.M.D. or D.D.S.).

Satisfactory completion of a residency program in an Oral and Maxillofacial Surgery approved by the American Dental Association (ADA) is an alternate pathway for prerequisite training for plastic surgery residency.

The satisfactory completion of this training **must** be verified in writing by the Oral and Maxillofacial Surgery program director. This program **may** include the integration of a medical school component resulting in a Doctor of Medicine (M.D.) degree or the Medical Degree may be obtained before or after residency training in Oral and Maxillofacial Surgery.

This combined training **must** also include a **minimum** of two years of **only** clinical general surgery training with progressive responsibility under the direction of the general surgery program director **after** obtaining the M.D. degree. These 24 months may be devoted only to those rotations in the 12 essential content areas of general surgery as listed on the previous page. The general surgery program director **must** verify, in writing, the completion of two years of clinical general surgery training, the levels of responsibility held, inclusive dates and specific month-by-month content of rotations **and evidence of current admissibility to the American Board of Oral and Maxillofacial Surgery Board examination process must be provided**. Rotations in general surgery during medical school prior to the M.D. degree will **not** be considered as fulfilling any part of the two-year minimum requirement. If the general surgery training is completed at an institution other than the sponsoring institution of the Oral and Maxillofacial

Surgery residency, then this training must be completed consecutively with both years spent in the same general surgery program which has been approved by the Residency Review Committee (RRC) for surgery and is accredited by the Accreditation Council for Graduate Medical Education (ACGME) in the United States.

VERIFICATION OF PREREQUISITE TRAINING

To obtain written verification from the program director under whom the resident completed prerequisite training, the Board Office will mail a **Verification Form** to the program director for completion and return to the Board Office. Residents should notify the Board Office when prerequisite training is completed. It is the resident's responsibility to determine that the form has been completed and returned to the Board Office.

REQUISITE TRAINING

GRADUATE EDUCATION IN PLASTIC SURGERY

A minimum of two years of plastic surgery training is required, and the final year must be at the senior level. Residents entering a plastic surgery residency accredited for three years of training must complete the entire three years, including one year of senior responsibility.

Residents may transfer, prior to the last two years, from an Independent Program to another Independent Program and from an Integrated Program to another Integrated Program, but they **may not** exchange accredited years of training between the two different models without prior approval by The American Board of Plastic Surgery Inc. **and** the Residency Review Committee for Plastic Surgery. Residents must request any anticipated transfers in writing and obtain prior approval by the Board well in advance of the proposed change in program. Refer to the transfer to Integrated Programs found later in this booklet.

Residents are required to complete **both years** of a two-year program in the **same** institution or the **last two** years of a three-year program in the **same** institution. In either instance, the final year must be at the senior level.

It is imperative that residents hold positions of increasing responsibility when obtaining training in more than one institution, and one full year of experience must be at the senior level. The normal training year for the program must be completed. No credit is granted for a partial year of training.

Training in plastic surgery must be obtained in either the United States or Canada. The Board recognizes training in those programs in the United States that have been approved by the Residency Review Committee (RRC-PS) for Plastic Surgery and accredited by the Accreditation Council for Graduate Medical Education (ACGME) or those programs approved by the Royal College of Physicians and Surgeons of Canada (RCPSC).

CONTENT OF TRAINING

Residents must hold positions of increasing responsibility for the care of patients during these years of training. For this reason, major operative experience and senior responsibility are essential to surgical education and training.

An important factor in the development of a surgeon is an opportunity to grow, under guidance and supervision, by progressive and successive stages to eventually assume complete responsibility for the surgical care of the patient.

The Board considers a residency in plastic surgery to be a full-time endeavor and looks with disfavor upon any other arrangement. The minimal acceptable training year is 48 weeks. Should absence exceed four weeks per annum for any reason, the circumstances and possible make-up

> time of this irregular training arrangement must be approved by the program director and the additional months required in the program must be approved by the Residency Review Committee (RRC-PS) for Plastic Surgery and documentation of this approval must be provided to the Board by the program director. No credit but no penalty is given for military, maternity/paternity or other leaves during training." (I know that was painful; you've had enough.)

WHAT THIS MEANS is that in order to sit for board certification, you are required to fulfill a minimum of three years of general surgery and two years of plastic surgery. I, on the other hand, had done much more during my training, and for that I am immensely proud. I completed five, not three, years of general surgery training at Lenox Hill Hospital, the Cornell University affiliate at the time. In my fifth year I served as administrative chief resident. Lenox Hill Hospital's training program in general surgery is a pyramid program. That means, it is competitive all along the way. It begins with 12 interns but ends with only two chief residents; meaning that people are excluded from the program each year based on performance. Only two people get to complete the residency program.

From Lenox Hill Hospital, I went on to plastic surgery training at the University of Michigan. There I completed two years of plastic surgery training at one of the best programs in the country. I also served as administrative chief resident at that program.

I could have been done at that point, but chose to do more. I wasn't satisfied with the minimum. I knew I wanted to do aesthetic or cosmetic surgery, and Dr. Timothy Miller, a professor at UCLA School of Medicine, was starting a fellowship in aesthetic plastic surgery.

This is where it gets interesting and it is here where Harvey either missed the boat, was too lazy to do the research, or just plain stupid. There are four areas of plastic surgery: 1) craniofacial surgery which involves moving bones around in the face, and pertains to anatomic defects in children and accident victims; 2) hand surgery, which is self-explanatory; 3) reconstructive surgery, which has to do with moving flaps around to cover holes or loss of tissue; and 4) aesthetic or cosmetic surgery.

Cosmetic surgery is actually a small part of what plastic surgeons do, but as a result of its relationship to Hollywood and movie stars, gets the majority of the press. In fact, in the plastic surgery community, programs are deemed better if they virtually ignore vanity surgery and concentrate on the more advanced techniques in reconstructive surgery including bone growth and microsurgical techniques. As a result, residents don't get a lot of cosmetic surgery training, and that's another reason why I chose to extend my training to include a fellowship in aesthetic surgery.

This is a fact that board certified plastic surgeons don't want you to know. They don't want you to know that you can be board certified and have never done a face lift, a tummy tuck, or a breast augmentation on your own. It is simply a cheap advertising tool that suggests an air of expertise but guarantees nothing. I am particularly sensitive to it because when I started my fellowship in aesthetic surgery at UCLA, it was precisely that group of board certified casual faculty who began to dismantle the aesthetic fellowship. And you want to know why? Because they make most of their money doing cosmetic surgery, and the last thing they needed was to produce a lot of Dr. Adams. The last thing they needed was to produce cosmetic surgeons with more training than they have.

They weren't about to let better trained aesthetic surgeons enter the market. And so Harvey Levin emerged as the naïve clown because he missed the real story. He failed to see that they hate and resent surgeons like me because I am better trained and refuse to join their club. Mr. Levin helped them continue to fool the public. Dr. West knew this. She was an extremely smart and educated woman who interviewed a number of physicians (according to the coroner's report) before deciding on Dr. Adams. In fact, all my patients know this. As lead dog, Harvey missed it and then led the pack, including the real news reporters, down the wrong path. The real story here is not board certification. The real story is why this program is no longer offered at UCLA even though the other three areas of plastic surgery offer fellowships.

Now board certification is important, and I would advise any resident to pursue it. It's not that it means that much if you have it, but if you don't, they will surely one day find a way to use it against you. I knew that day would come and I wanted it. I wanted people to talk about training and expertise, not advertising.

However, approximately three years ago one of my closest friends, Dr. Noel Tenenbaum, an excellent plastic surgeon in Tampa, Florida, challenged me to take it. "Okay," he said, "You've made your point. Get it done."

And so, I got on a plane and flew to Chicago for a review course. The problem was, when I got off the plane, I collapsed with bilateral pulmonary emboli and required two weeks of hospitalization. It would appear that God laughs at those who make plans, because God has his own plans. It would appear that God wanted you and me, Mr. Levin to come together so that we could make clear an issue that needed to be clarified. So let's review:

Dr. Adams attended and graduated from Harvard College, which is ranked number one in the country by *US News* as America's best college (now, I know some of my best friends who attended Princeton would argue that at the time they attended Princeton it was ranked #1—but let's just say I chose Harvard over Princeton). I then went on to Ohio State University College of Medicine, ranked 37th out of 116 of America's best graduate schools. I then trained in general surgery at Lenox Hill Hospital, the Cornell affiliate, ranked 15th; plastic surgery at the University of Michigan, ranked 10th; and UCLA for aesthetic surgery, ranked 13th. My point is not to impress you. My point is to impress upon you that there are different ways of going about medical training, each of which carries its own advantages. I chose not to do the minimum. And think about it. Where would we be if everybody settled for the minimum? Where would Tiger Woods be as a golfer if he did just the minimum? Where would George Clooney, Brad Pitt, Sam Jackson, and Denzel Washington be as actors if they just did the minimum? Where would Spike Lee or Steven Spielberg be as directors if they did just the minimum? And where would America be as a country if we did just the minimum?

Now don't get me wrong. I'm not suggesting that the ability to do cosmetic surgery is merely a function of the number of years of training. Nonetheless, the question placed on the table by the media was really, who is in fact qualified to do it? I would make the argument that there are other disciplines besides plastic surgery that also do a good job at cosmetic surgery. (Understand, cosmetic surgery isn't specifically a discipline. It merely refers to aesthetic procedures.) There is absolutely no doubt whatsoever in my mind that there are gynecologists who do better liposuction. There are general surgeons who do better tummy tucks and breasts. There are ophthalmologists who do better eyelid surgery. There are otolaryngologists who do better noses and face lifts.

The point I'm trying to make is that when a surgeon says, "I'm board certified" in a certain area, what he is really saying, if you scratch him hard enough, is that "this is my area and I don't want anyone infringing on it." But the truth of the matter is that this is still America, and America is about competition. So I say, let the cream rise to the top. Those people who are good at it will attract the clientele who will follow them. The notion that this procedure is mine exclusively, the notion of restraint of trade, is not only anti-American—we solved that in 1938 with the passing of the Taft-Hartley Act-it's just plain wrong. (And by the way, for the skeptics, I'm still eligible for the boards, I simply choose not to join their club and therefore, be a party to the discrimination I see them shell out every day. Watch a board certified Plastic surgeon talk training as if he or she has it. Then ask him if he does eyelid surgery. If he says yes ask him why? Shouldn't only ophthalmologists' do eyelid surgery? Ask any otolaryngologist about nose surgery. I never saw it as us versus them. It would seem to me the only person important is the patient.)

Jan Adams

From: Michael Moore [mmoore@dataharborsolutions.com]
Sent: Friday, January 11, 2008 2:40 PM
To: Michael D Moore
Subject: AMERICAN BOARD OF PLASTIC SURGERY 2008 Written Examination On-line Reply Form

Today you have been mailed (via U.S. Mail) information regarding the 2008 Written Examination On-line Reply Form. Instructions for logging in to the Board's website and your Board Number will be included in this mailing. Once you receive the packet you can log in to the Board's website to complete and finalize the Reply Form by the deadline March 3, 2008.

Please contact the Board Office at 215-587-9322 should you have any questions.
* *
For technical support, please contact Web Data Solutions at 312-944-0642 or support@dataharborsolutions.com <mailto:support@dataharborsolutions.com>.

Figure 7

3

I SHARED WITH YOU EARLIER HOW THE PRESS HATES A VACUUM. I would not break the law and, more importantly, violate my patient's confidentiality by sharing privileged information, and so the press began to create stories on their own to fill that hour or complete that column.

The story got increasingly away from the issue at hand—the death of Dr. West—and more and more malicious concerning me in an attempt to draw me out. So don't be fooled—the media was looking for a story, but frankly too lazy or too stupid to see them. The problem was they had plenty of stories out there. They simply chose to ignore them, returning instead to their tabloid levels of misguided high-tech information age lynching.

They could have investigated a number of issues surrounding plastic surgery: the nature of informed consent, unrealistic expectations on the part of a patient, the inherent risk of surgery or anesthesia, and many others, including malpractice suits. Instead, they chose to expose issues that were already public record. But even then—and this is what's important to understand—they presented only half the story.

Dr. Adams, they wrote, had more than one DUI arrest and their goal was to suggest alcoholism. No one said it because all media companies have fulltime lawyers on staff whose job it is to make certain they don't step over the line. And so, they all have become adept at innuendo, but not at facts. The data did not support that conclusion so they only told half the story.

I did have the two run-ins with the police to which Mr. Levin refers. There was also alleged alcohol abuse in both. But don't let me tell the story, let's first let the authorities tell it from their perspective:

MAY-18-2007 13:55 ATTORNEY GENERAL LA 213 897 9395 P.02

FILED
STATE OF CALIFORNIA
MEDICAL BOARD OF CALIFORNIA
SACRAMENTO April 10 2007
BY: M. [signature] **ANALYST**

EDMUND G. BROWN JR., Attorney General
of the State of California
PAUL C. AMENT
Supervising Deputy Attorney General
RICHARD D. MARINO, State Bar No. 90471
Deputy Attorney General
California Department of Justice
300 S. Spring Street, Suite 1702
Los Angeles, California 90013
Telephone: (213) 897-8644
Facsimile: (213) 897-9395
E-mail: richard.marino@doj.ca.gov

Attorneys for Complainant

BEFORE THE
DIVISION OF MEDICAL QUALITY
MEDICAL BOARD OF CALIFORNIA
DEPARTMENT OF CONSUMER AFFAIRS
STATE OF CALIFORNIA

In the Matter of the Accusation Against:	Case No. 17-2006-175650
JAN ADAMS, M.D. 553 Emerald Way Laguna Beach, California 92551	**ACCUSATION**
Physician and Surgeon's Certificate No. A51004,	
Respondent.	

Complainant alleges:

PARTIES

1. David T. Thornton (Complainant) brings this Accusation solely in his official capacity as the Executive Director of the Medical Board of California (Board).

2. On or about July 23, 1992, the Board issued Physician and Surgeon's Certificate Number A51004 to Jan Adams, M.D. (Respondent.) Unless renewed, this license will expire on April 30, 2008.

JURISDICTION

3. This Accusation is brought before the Board's Division of Medical Quality under the authority of the following laws. All section references are to the Business and Professions Code unless otherwise indicated.

1

Figure 8

MAY-18-2007 13:55 ATTORNEY GENERAL LA 213 897 9395 P.03

A. Section 2227 of the Code provides that a licensee who is found guilty under the Medical Practice Act may have his or her license revoked, suspended for a period not to exceed one year, placed on probation and required to pay the costs of probation monitoring, or such other action taken in relation to discipline as the Division deems proper.

B. Section 2234 of the Code, in pertinent part, provides:

"The Division of Medical Quality shall take action against any licensee who is charged with unprofessional conduct. In addition to other provisions of this article, unprofessional conduct includes, but is not limited to, the following:

"(a) Violating or attempting to violate, directly or indirectly, assisting in or abetting the violation of, or conspiring to violate any provision of this chapter [Chapter 5, the Medical Practice Act].

". . .

"(f) Any action or conduct which would have warranted the denial of a certificate."

C. Section 2239 of the Code provides:

"(a) The use or prescribing for or administering to himself or herself, of any controlled substance; or the use of any of the dangerous drugs specified in Section 4022, or of alcoholic beverages, to the extent, or in such a manner as to be dangerous or injurious to the licensee, or to any other person or to the public, or to the extent that such use impairs the ability of the licensee to practice medicine safely or more than one misdemeanor or any felony involving the use, consumption, or self-administration of any of the substances referred to in this section, or any combination thereof, constitutes unprofessional conduct. The record of the conviction is conclusive evidence of such unprofessional conduct.

"(b) A plea or verdict of guilty or a conviction following a plea of nolo contendere is deemed to be a conviction within the meaning of this section. The Division of Medical Quality may order discipline of the licensee in

2

Figure 8 (continued)

MAY-18-2007 13:56 ATTORNEY GENERAL LA 213 897 9395 P.04

accordance with Section 2227 or the Division of Licensing may order the denial of the license when the time for appeal has elapsed or the judgment of conviction has been affirmed on appeal or when an order granting probation is made suspending imposition of sentence, irrespective of a subsequent order under the provisions of Section 1203.4 of the Penal Code allowing such person to withdraw his or her plea of guilty and to enter a plea of not guilty, or setting aside the verdict of guilty, or dismissing the accusation, complaint, information, or indictment."

FIRST CAUSE FOR DISCIPLINE

(Multiple Criminal Convictions For Alcohol-Related Offenses)

4. Respondent's Physician and Surgeon's Certificate is subject to disciplinary action pursuant to Business and Professions Code section 2239 in that Respondent has sustained multiple convictions for alcohol-related offenses, as follows:

December 21, 2006

A. On or about March 31, 2006, at approximately 2:32 a.m., members of the California Highway Patrol (CHP) observed Respondent driving eastbound in excess of the posted speed limit along Interstate 10 (Santa Monica Freeway), near the La Brea Avenue exit. The CHP officers made a traffic stop at which time they found that Respondent was driving without a valid California driver's license and observed the strong odor of alcohol emanating from Respondent and his vehicle. Respondent was administered a series of field sobriety tests which he did not complete successfully. Respondent was transported to the Central Los Angeles CHP office where he underwent two breath analyzer tests. Each test showed a blood alcohol level of .10 percent. Respondent was arrested for driving under the influence of alcohol, in violation of Vehicle Code section 23152, subdivision (a), a misdemeanor.

B. On or about April 4, 2006, in the case entitled *People of the State of California v. Jan Rudalgo Adams*, Los Angeles County Superior Court

3

Figure 8 (continued)

Case No. 6MP03940, Respondent was charged with driving under the influence of alcohol or drugs, in violation of Vehicle Code section 23152, subdivision (a), a misdemeanor (Count 1); driving with a blood alcohol level of .08 percent or greater, in violation of Vehicle Code section 23152, subdivision (b) (Count 2); and, driving with a suspended license, in violation of Vehicle Code section 14601.1, subdivision (a), a misdemeanor.

C. On or about May 10, 2006, Respondent entered not guilty pleas to each of the charged offenses. The matter was set for trial.

D. On or about October 25, 2006, Respondent withdrew his previously entered not guilty plea to the charge alleged in Count 3–namely, driving with a suspended license–and entered a plea of *nolo contendere*. Adjudication of the remaining charges proceeded to jury trial.

E. On or about November 11, 2006, the jury found Respondent not guilty of the charge alleged in Count 1–namely, driving under the influence of alcohol or drugs and guilty of the charge alleged in Count 2–namely, driving with a blood alcohol level of .08 percent or greater.

F. On or about December 21, 2006, proceedings were suspended. Respondent was placed on probation for five years with the following terms and conditions, among others: serve 96 hours in the Los Angeles County Jail; perform 45 days of Cal Trans service; participate in the 18 month alcohol treatment and counseling program; enroll in the SB-38 program; and attend 60 Alcoholics Anonymous meetings at the minimum rate of two meetings each week.

May 9, 2003

G. On or about January 16, 2003, in the matter entitled *People of the State of California v. Jan Rudolgo Adams*, Los Angeles County Superior Court Number 3WL00123, Respondent was charged with driving under the influence of alcohol or drugs, in violation of Vehicle Code section 23152, a

Figure 8 (continued)

MAY-18-2007 13:56 ATTORNEY GENERAL LA 213 897 9395 P.06

misdemeanor.[1]

H. On or about February 27, 2003, Respondent entered a plea of not guilty and the matter was set for trial.

I. On or about May 9, 2003, Respondent withdrew his pleas of not guilty and entered a plea of *nolo contendere*. Proceedings were suspended and Respondent was placed on probation for three years with the following terms and conditions, among others: 1) that he complete the three month first offender alcohol and drug education and counseling program; 2) that for 90 days he only drive to and from work; and, 3) that he not drive without a valid California driver's license.

SECOND CAUSE FOR DISCIPLINE

(Use of Alcohol)

5. Respondent's Physician and Surgeon's Certificate is subject to disciplinary action in that Respondent has used alcohol to the extent or in such a manner as to be dangerous or injurious to himself and others within the meaning of Business and Professions Code section 2239, as follows:

A. Complainant refers to and, by this reference, incorporates herein Paragraph 4, above, as though fully set forth.

THIRD CAUSE FOR DISCIPLINE

(Unprofessional Conduct)

6. Respondent's Physician and Surgeon's Certificate is subject to disciplinary action in that Respondent has engaged in unprofessional conduct, in violation of Business and Professions Code section 2234, generally, as follows:

A. Complainant refers to and, by this reference, incorporates

---

1. Respondent was arrested for this offense on September 6, 2002. On that date, Respondent lost control of his vehicle and struck a parked car. Respondent told law enforcement officers and others that he lost control of his car when another vehicle failed to stop for a traffic signal. Respondent did not provide a description of the vehicle.

5

Figure 8 (continued)

MAY-18-2007 13:57 ATTORNEY GENERAL LA 213 897 9395 P.07

herein Paragraph 4, above, as though fully set forth.

PRAYER

WHEREFORE, Complainant requests that a hearing be held on the matters herein alleged, and that following the hearing, the Medical Board of California issue a decision:

1. Revoking or suspending Physician and Surgeon's Certificate Number A51004, issued to Jan Adams, M.D.

2. Revoking, suspending or denying approval of Jan Adams's authority to supervise physician's assistants, pursuant to section 3527 of the Code;

3. Ordering Jan Adams, M.D., if placed on probation, to pay the Medical Board of California the costs of probation monitoring; and,

4 Taking such other and further action as deemed necessary and proper.

DATED: April 10, 2007

DAVID T. THORNTON
Executive Director
Medical Board of California
State of California

Complainant

LA2006504285

50141198.wpd

6

TOTAL P.07

Figure 8 (continued)

Firstly, it was around 1:30 a.m. on March 31, 2006, when I was pulled over for speeding, not 2:30 a.m. but we will allow them that. Secondly, further check by the District attorney's office demonstrated that my license was indeed valid and that charge was dismissed. Thirdly, the testimony of the arresting officer during the trial contradicts the statement "Respondent was administered a series of field sobriety tests which he did not complete successfully." In fact, the arresting officer, CHP officer McNurlin, testifies, under oath, during the trial that following completion of the sobriety tests, she did not believe I was under the influence. That is why on page 4, line 13, paragraph E of the Medical Board's Accusation "the jury found Respondent not guilty of the charge alleged in Count 1-namely, driving under the influence of alcohol or drugs".

The Accusation goes on to say that the "Respondent was transported to the Central Los Angeles CHP office where he underwent two breath analyzer tests". This could not be further from the truth, and frankly, has served as a source of friction between me and my attorney Thomas Byrne. Tom is gentleman who I like a great deal. Tom wanted to win this case. I wanted to tell the truth. Tom was concerned about the jury. I wanted to tell the truth.

The officers involved didn't take me to the station. They put me in the backseat and went to pick up another DUI suspect, a Latin fellow.

During the trial, the arresting officers both testified that they administered a portable field breath analyzer and that is what prompted them to arrest me. The problem is they never administered that test. (And that is what prompted me to take this case to trial.) While one was administering the field sobriety test, the other, a white male, stood approximately ten yards away observing me. He got a call on his car radio and walked over to answer it. He came back, whispered in the female officer's ear, she abruptly ended the field sobriety test and away we went to pick up this other fellow.

After their evaluation of him, we all went inside the CHP office. I phrase it that way because oddly enough, they picked this guy up on the corner right outside the gate to the CHP parking lot.

I did have the breath analyzer test at this time, approximately one and a half hours after being stopped for speeding. I did blow .09 and .10 on successive tries.

A prior incident occurred in March, 2003. The Medical Board's Accusation oddly omits the particulars and only mentions the disposition. I have no explanation for that, I only make the observation.

While parking my car in front of my apartment complex I bumped the car in front of me. Frankly, I was sleepy and was not paying attention and was distracted by the headlights of a car that turned right on a red light behind me as I pulled into the space. Examination demonstrated some damage to my bumper but no obvious problem with the other car. At any rate I put in a call to the UCLA campus police to get a police report for insurance purposes. The UCLA police arrived, but informed me that we would have to wait for LAPD because where I was parked was out of their jurisdiction.

Approximately one hour later the LAPD arrived and as I explained to them what had happened, the owner of the car in front of me arrived. We examined his car and he informed us that the bumper looked pushed in a bit and that there was a scratch on the bumper. Apparently, the car's owner suggested to the police officer that "he thought he smelled alcohol", because following that the officer asked if I would perform a field sobriety test.

I made it clear to him that I had not been drinking and that I had been sitting here talking with the officers from UCLAPD for an hour and none of them had suggested that. He insisted on the test, but I suggested we go to the station and use the breath analyzer.

We did. I blew into the analyzer five times-that's right five times-and no alcohol was detected.

The officer then called a supervisor, a black female sergeant, who informed me that I would need a blood test or that they would treat it as a refusal. She was fair, and I explained to her that I had not refused. I had blown into the machine five times. I had told the officer from the start that I had not been drinking and I wasn't taking a blood test because this was stupid.

At trial I pleaded no contest. I also reported this case to the Medical Board of California back in 2003, they investigated it, and dismissed any action (that is, until now). (By the way, the owner of the car turned out to be a bartender at a restaurant around the corner from my apartment, maybe that's why he smelled alcohol.)

Now, don't get me wrong—drinking and driving is stupid and without a doubt the incorrect thing to do. I personally solved it by simply not drinking. But there is a larger issue here, and that is worth discussing. The Constitution of the United States is designed to protect citizens from—get this—the government. And that, my friend, was a very wise thing. Understand that the largest money maker in America isn't General Motors or U.S. Steel or Exxon Oil—it's the criminal justice system. And in America, they are in the business of creating criminals. California law convicts you of a DUI if your blood alcohol level is greater than .08. I blew .09 and .1. That is hardly impressive as people have been known to blow up to .3 and .35 and still be awake. I tell you this because here's what's interesting. The State of California wants to lower the legal content to .05, and I see no sense in that. At .05, you only convict the housewife who is out having a glass of wine with her girlfriends at lunch. Any person trained in alcohol treatment will tell you that the chronic drinker or the problem drinker who blows 1.5 to 2.0 is probably on his way out, not in. So .05 doesn't get the problem drinker—it gets the housewife having lunch. Now, once again, I'm not suggesting that it's correct to drink and drive. As I said earlier, I've simply chosen not to participate in that game.

I'm saying the government is hypocritical in that if we do not want drinking and driving, have zero tolerance, not .05, not .08. Don't have people playing Russian roulette with whether they had one beer or two, or one cocktail or one glass of wine. Just make the law say, we have zero tolerance, don't do it, and then we won't have to worry about it.

Unfortunately though, as a physician, there is something even more sinister going on here. It's the Medical Board itself. You would think that a state agency, like the Medical Board, acting as a final adjudicator would be held to the same standard of impartiality as a judge. However, because it also conducts the investigation, the Board is really in partnership with the prosecutor (the attorney general). Having therefore made the determination to proceed with a hearing, the Board now has a stake in the outcome. They can't be objective about witnesses or testimony because the "facts" are obtained through the Board's own investigation by the Board's own investigators.

Let me show you what I mean. After the second interaction with the police, I decided to take a cold hard look at myself. My friend, Wynn Katz, thought I had gone completely crazy. I argued that before I chalk this up to the police harassing another black guy driving around Beverly Hills at night I would look at myself.

I contacted the Medical Board of California Diversion Program Services, told them my situation, and arranged for an interview. I met in Diamond Bar, California, with a Mr. Bernard Karmatz, M.S., LMFT. We filled out the necessary paper work and I consented to their agreement during the evaluation process.

I also received confirmation of our meeting from Mr. Karmatz. (Yet, from the beginning, there were already shenanigans going on. If you look at the Agreement, During Evaluation Process, Self-Referral you see that it is dated 12/14/06. However, Mr. Karmatz's Personal and Confidential letter is dated October, 10, 2006. At first I thought this was an innocent mistake but Mr. Karmatz, over time, proved himself to be less than genuine.

He goes on to say that he had "reviewed the case with Diversion Administration in Sacramento" and "they are directing" me "to stop your medical practice by the end of the regular business day on December 15, 2006". None of that was true. It was Mr. Karmatz acting independently.)

AGREEMENT
DURING EVALUATION PROCESS
Self-Referral

I, Jan Adams JRA M.D., am applying for admission to the Physician Diversion Program, a rehabilitation and monitoring program administered by the Division of Medical Quality of the Medical Board of California (MBC). I recognize that I may have a substance-related disorder or mental health-related disorder. I will be scheduled to meet with a Diversion Evaluation Committee for it to evaluate my particular circumstances, to determine if I am appropriate for, and will benefit from, the Diversion Program, and to finalize the treatment plan provisions of my Diversion Agreement.

I understand the Diversion Program's first priority is protecting the public's safety and welfare. I also understand that the Diversion Program is responsible for assisting and guiding me in my rehabilitation/recovery process. The purpose of this document is to explain the terms and conditions during the evaluation process.

I Jan Adams, M.D., agree to comply with the terms and conditions outlined below, pending a decision on whether I will be accepted into the Diversion Program:

JRA 1) I agree to restrict or cease my practice of medicine if the Diversion Program determines that I am impaired. Impairment may be determined by:

1) Practicing while under the influence of alcohol or other drugs.
2) Submitting a biological fluid test that results in a positive drug screen.
3) Refusing to submit to biological fluid testing.
4) Attending diversion group while under the influence of alcohol or drugs.
5) Documented reports from my work site monitor of unsafe practice performance.
6) Non-compliance with these Terms and Conditions.

JRA 2) I will enter a treatment program within one to seven days as directed if it is determined by the Diversion Program that treatment is necessary in order for me to practice medicine safely. The cost will be at my expense.

JRA 3) I will attend <u>one/two</u> facilitated Diversion Group meetings per week as directed, at the assigned location. If I am unable to attend, I will report the reason to the group facilitator and my Diversion Program case manager. I agree to stay current with group fees or make payment arrangements with the group facilitator. I will request Diversion Program approval prior to taking any time off from group. I will make up all missed Diversion Group meetings within the following week by attending Recovery Support Group meetings, such as Alcoholics Anonymous or Narcotics Anonymous, with my case manager's approval.

G:\Diversi\1 Office\2 Case Manager Templates\SelfReferralEvalAgrmntDrftw.wpd (6-22-99)

Figure 9

SELF-REFERRAL
PAGE 2

4) I will attend 7 Recovery Support Group Meetings, such as Alcoholics Anonymous or Narcotics Anonymous, per week as directed.

5) If directed by the Diversion Program, I will undergo a substance-related disorder and/or psychiatric evaluation if I have not had treatment for my condition. The cost will be at my expense.

6) I will abstain from the use of alcohol and all psychotropic drugs except those prescribed for me by another physician and approved by the Diversion Program.

7) I will report by telephone to my Diversion Program case manager all personal use of prescription drugs and the name of the prescribing physician. I will obtain a copy of all prescriptions written for me prior to having them filled. These copies will be given to my case manager.

8) I will not self-prescribe any medications which require a prescription.

9) I will provide a minimum of two observed biological fluid samples per month, as requested. The laboratory results of these tests will be submitted to the Diversion Program. The urine test lab fee and collection fee will be paid at the time of the testing. All fees are my responsibility.

10) I will obey all federal, state and local laws and rules governing the practice of medicine in the State of California. I will immediately report by telephone to my Diversion Program case manager any arrest or conviction of any offense.

11) I will immediately report by telephone to my Diversion Program case manager any relapse or use of alcohol or unauthorized drugs.

12) I understand and agree that my participation in the Diversion Program does not affect, alter, or curtail in any manner the MBC's authority to investigate and take disciplinary action against my license for any unprofessional conduct committed by me whether before, during, or after my participation in the Diversion Program.

13) Any expenses related to the requirements of the Diversion Program are my responsibility. I understand that any expenses incurred in my treatment (i.e., hospitalization, biological fluid analysis, doctor fees, meeting fees, etc.) are my responsibility. I understand that payment of fees is to be kept current or payment arrangements made.

G:\Diversion Office\2 Case Manager Templates\SelfReferralAgmntDrftw.wpd (6-22-99)

Figure 9 (continued)

SELF-REFERRAL
PAGE 3

14) Other provisions -

I have read and discussed this document with the Diversion Program case manager. I understand and agree to the Terms and Conditions outlined above and I acknowledge receipt of a copy of this document.

12-14-06 Date
Applicant Signature

Bernie Karmatz, MFT 12-14/06 Date
Diversion Program Case Manager

Date
Diversion Program Administrator

G:\Diversi\1Office\2 Case Manager Templates\SelfReferralEvalAgrmntDrftw.wpd (6-22-99)

Figure 9 (continued)

STATE OF CALIFORNIA-STATE AND CONSUMER SERVICES AGENCY — ARNOLD SCHWARZENEGGER, Governor

State of California Department of Consumer Affairs

MEDICAL BOARD OF CALIFORNIA
Diversion Program Services
1370 S. VALLEY VISTA DRIVE, SUITE 240
DIAMOND BAR, CA 91765-3923
(909) 396 5311 909) 860 - 7480 (FAX)

Personal and Confidential

October 10, 2006

Jan Rudalgo Adams, M.D.
553 Emerald Bay
Laguna Beach, California 92651

Dear Dr. Adams,

Thank you for your participation in the initial interview today and agreeing to participate in the Diversion Program. I have reviewed your case with the Diversion Administration in Sacramento. They are directing you to stop your medical practice by the end of the regular business day on December 15, 2006. As discussed today, you are encouraged to review this situation with peers in the Diversion Group this evening.

You are to proceed to contact and arrange for, an initial evaluation at one of the three approved treatment facilities noted in this letter. You are to contact me immediately if you are not able to enter one of these facilities for this initial assessment by December 20, 2006. Each treatment facility will determine the number of days necessary to complete this required assessment, which will address whether a residential program for alcohol abuse is indicated.

The treatment facilities you are to contact are the Hazelden Springbrook facility in Newberg, Oregon. Contact the Assessment Coordinator, Ashley Burrows at 800 - 257 - 7800, Ext 4446. The additional facilities you may contact are Talbott Recovery program in Atlanta, Georgia (800 - 445 - 4232), and the William J. Farley Center in Williamsburg, Virginia. The Coordinator for the Farley Center is Arnie Zepel, who may be contacted at 619 -587 - 2725.

Sincerely,

Bernard Karmatz, M.S., LMFT
Diversion Program Case Manager

cc. file

Figure 10

Nonetheless, I did go to Hazelden Springbrook facility in Newberg, Oregon for evaluation. I was admitted on 1/07/07 and discharged on 1/10/07. It was one of the most invasive ordeals I have ever encountered. A counselor brings you in and instructs you in what will take place and assures you that the entire process is strictly confidential. A nurse then conducts a history and physical exam and assures you that the process is strictly confidential. Another counselor then arrives who searches your belongings for contraband and assures you that the process is strictly confidential. Finally you meet your personal counselor who informs you that the process is strictly confidential, but that she can't get started until you give her a list of ten people to contact in order to substantiate the information you give her.

Its then off to evaluations by a psychiatrist, a psychologist, a social worker, and finally the individual who administers psychological tests including personality tests, tests for depression, and basic verbal and coordination tests.

I was discharged in three days because the experts concluded that my behaviors and my history did not meet the criteria for alcoholism or alcohol dependency. (It seems I am a knucklehead for having driven home after drinking with my friends, but that doesn't make me an alcoholic. So you would think that after hearing that Mr. Karmatz and the Medical Board of California would have, at least, softened their approach: No such luck.)

Before I had gotten off the plane from Newberg, Mr. Karmatz had scheduled me for admission to another facility. He hadn't even received the results from Hazelden yet (no one had because they had not been released) and over the phone, he was already trying to bully me. I calmly hanged- up on him and contacted his boss in Sacramento.

Mr. Frank Valine, the administrator in Sacramento, seemed reasonable. He advised me to take it easy. Acknowledged that the thing to do was wait on Hazelden's report and offered to discuss things once the report was out.

STATE OF CALIFORNIA-STATE AND CONSUMER SERVICES AGENCY ARNOLD SCHWARZENEGGER, Governor

State of California Department of Consumer Affairs

MEDICAL BOARD OF CALIFORNIA
Diversion Program Services
1370 S. VALLEY VISTA DRIVE, SUITE 240
DIAMOND BAR, CA 91765-3923
(909) 396 5311 909) 860 - 7480 (FAX)

Personal and Confidential

January 16, 2007

Jan Rudalgo Adams, M.D.
553 Emerald Bay
Laguna Beach, California 92651

Dear Dr. Adams,

As a result of our telephone conversation today, I am documenting my request of January 11, 2007 for you to contact the Cornerstone program. The telephone numbers are (800) 385 - 9889 or (714) 730 - 5399. You should request to speak with Bonnie McClain, Alternative Sentencing Coordinator, and complete an intake interview. This is based upon your current legal status, the DSM IV, Axis I, diagnosis of Alcohol Abuse and Axis II issues. Currently, you cannot be scheduled for a Diversion Evaluation Committee meeting.

In accord with the Diversion Agreement, please continue to remain off work, and attending seven designated support groups, including not less than five AA meetings. You may also benefit from a CODA group and an anger management group. Please use the enclosed attendance cards to provide evidence of compliance.

Additionally, please provide the previously requested information regarding your work site monitor, including the address where the monitor would prefer to receive mail.

Contact me if there are any additional concerns.

Sincerely,

Bernard Karmatz, M.S., LMFT
Diversion Program Case Manager

cc: file
Marsha Vanover, Ph.D.

Figure 11

Still, I received a letter from Mr. Karmatz dated January 16, 2007. I would really like to go on about Mr. Karmatz's dishonesty and his manipulation of the system, but I'll let our series of letters speak for themselves:

Jan R. Adams M.D.

Personal and Confidential

January 19, 2007

Bernard Karmatz, M.S., LMFT
1370 S. Valley Vista Drive,Suite 240
Diamond Bar, CA 91765-3923

Dear Mr. Karmatz,

In response to your letter of January 16, 2007, I am documenting my response to your requests. You state that "...in accord with the Diversion Agreement, please continue to remain off work...". The Diversion Agreement states that " I agree to restrict or cease my Practice if the Diversion Program determines that I am Impaired. Impairment may be determined by:

1) Practicing while under the influence of alcohol or other drugs. (In my 15 years of practice, there has never been any complaint like that whatsoever. I sudmitted to you , Dr Raad Jeroudi, the owner, and daily anesthesiologist, who confirmed that he has worked daily with me and has never even remotely thought such a thing was going on. He further offered to you that there were 20 other people in the office and none of them had witnessed anything like that. He further went on to offer that " in fact, Dr Adams is the one we call if there is a problem because we know he will make himself available, and he has at varying times during the day and night.)
2) Submitting a biological fluid test that results in a positive drug screen. (I've done that since my self-referral to the program and have been consistent in complying and have not had a positive test.)
3) Refusing to submit to biological fluid testing. (I have made all tests, including taking the time to wait for the examiner when he was late.)
4) Attending diversion group while under the influence of alcohol or drugs. (I have certainly not violated that directive.)
5) Documented reports from my work site monitor of unsafe practice performance. (Again, I would refer you to item 1.)
6) Non-compliance with these Terms and Conditions. (I have done what you have directed me to do.)

Furthermore, I went to Hazelden for an evaluation. They determined that I did not meet theDSM IV criteria for alcohol dependency or alcoholism. Prior to going I asked you why Hazelden, why not some place in California? You said that their results were

Figure 12

consistent and in your experience they were the place you could rely on for consistent data. I reiterated that "you mean to tell me that no one in California can do this? With UCLA, San Francisco, SC, and San Diego, there is no other place who's results you trust? You said again, "we trust their opinions". And yet you attempted to schedule me for treatment before getting the results. The fact is you had made a determination without the necessary data, and now are trying propel me into a treatment program, for which your experts admit there is no disease.

You further went on to say that that is what Sacramento wanted, but you were unaware that I had talked with FrankValine prior to our conversation and he had said nothing of the sort. In fact he had suggested that I take it one day at a time, and let's wait for the report.

I then proceeded to Cornerstone and met with Bonnie McClain and Jan McClary. Following the interview, it was suggested that I think about what I wanted to do. The interviewer felt that without the diagnosis of alcohol dependency, she wasn't sure that any of the inpatient or outpatient programs were right for me, but that I might benefit from their educational programs, and further that they might be able to cater a program to what might be beneficial to me.

You further go on to inform me that I cannot be scheduled for a Diversion Evaluation Committee meeting but are unable to tell me what the requirements are for securing that meeting.

You also suggest that I might benefit from an anger management group, but I would suggest that asking you to substantiate your claims and recommendations does not make me angry. And unless you are prepared to substantiate that claim you should stop with the shoot-from-the-hip diagnoses. You tried to intimidate me with the statement that you believed "Marsha might think I'm an alcoholic", but your own experts at Hazelden have put that to rest. So stop with that.

I do truly look forward to working with you to resolve this matter. And, by the way, just because someone does not fit your paradigm, does not mean that they cannot benefit from your services. That is why I sought you out. Nevertheless, the validity of what you do must be judged by your willingness not to rubber stamp everyone. Indeed, if there is an air of thoughtfulness and fairness around what you do, I believe those individuals who otherwise might fall through the cracks, would seek you out.

Sincerely

Jan R. Adams M.D.

Figure 12 (continued)

Two weeks later Mr. Karmatz was at it again:

Jan 29 07 03:34p B.Karmatz,M.S., LMFT (909) 445 - 0374 p.1

STATE OF CALIFORNIA-STATE AND CONSUMER SERVICES AGENCY ARNOLD SCHWARZENEGGER, Governor

State of California Department of Consumer Affairs

MEDICAL BOARD OF CALIFORNIA
Diversion Program Services
1370 S. VALLEY VISTA DRIVE, SUITE 240
DIAMOND BAR, CA 91765-3923
(909) 396 5311 909) 860 - 7480 (FAX)

Personal and Confidential

January 29, 2007

Jan Rudalgo Adams, M.D.
553 Emerald Bay
Laguna Beach, California 92651

Dear Dr. Adams,

Please be advised that there was a diluted U A test result reported on January 11, 2007 from a specimen you submitted on January 5, 2007. Please fax or e mail an explanation of this result. Generally, you are requested to refrain from consuming liquids two hours prior to a test which may cause a dilute result.

Please contact me if there are any additional questions.

Sincerely,

Bernard Karmatz MS

Bernard Karmatz, M.S., LMFT
Diversion Program Case Manager

cc: file

Figure 13

This prompted another even more ridiculous response from me.

Jan R. Adams M.D.

January 29, 2007

Bernard Karmatz, M.S.,LMFT
Diversion Program Case Manager
1370 S. Valley Vista Drive
Suite 240
Diamond Bar, CA 91765

Dear Mr. Karmatz,

Thank you for advising me that " there was a diluted U A test result reported on January 11, 2007 from a specimen (you) submitted on January 5, 2007". I'm not sure I need to offer you "an explanation of this result" since you so eloquently point out that "generally, you are requested to refrain from consuming liquids two hours prior to a test which may cause a dilute result".

I am, however, going to take your failure to comment on either alcohol or ethyl glucuronide to mean none was present. After all, the purpose of the test, that is, the purpose of urine monitoring, is to prevent, or to provide early warning of, relapse. Nevertheless, since your experts at Hazelden were unable to arrive at a diagnosis of alcohol dependency, or alcoholism, there is nothing to relapse to.

The real issue here is that if drinking water prior to the test creates problems, then I will refrain from doing that. Nevertheless, I don't need your sarcasm of "an explanation of this result" in order to do that. Simply communicate to me what you need me to do and I will do it. Just lose the extracurricular remarks. Once again, just because someone doesn't fit your paradigm, doesn't mean they can't benefit from your services.

Let's you and I demonstrate to others out there that there is an air of fairness and respect surrounding diversion that makes it safe for them to seek help.

Sincerely,

Jan R. Adams M.D.

cc: Tom Byrne, Esq
Henry Fenton, Esq
Marsha Vanover, Phd
Frank Valine, Director, Diversion Program

Figure 14

But, our Mr. Karmatz is relentless. Three to four weeks later I received another letter from him. Again he referred to some unverifiable administrative review and requested once again that I begin the program at Cornerstone.

02/21/2007 17:10 9093965313 *MED BOARD-DBDO* PAGE 01

STATE OF CALIFORNIA-STATE AND CONSUMER SERVICES AGENCY ARNOLD SCHWARZENEGGER, Governor

State of California Department of Consumer Affairs

MEDICAL BOARD OF CALIFORNIA
Diversion Program Services
1370 S. VALLEY VISTA DRIVE, SUITE 240
DIAMOND BAR, CA 91765-3923
(909) 396 6311 909) 860 - 7480 (FAX)

<u>Personal and Confidential</u>

February 21, 2007

Jan Rudalgo Adams, M.D.
553 Emerald Bay
Laguna Beach, California 92651

Dear Dr. Adams,

Please be advised that after Administrative review, you are requested to begin the outpatient program at the Cornerstone facility this week, and comply with the terms of the Diversion Agreement, which you signed on December 14, 2006. At this time, it is not known what the length of the outpatient program will be. You are expected to be in the Diversion Group each Monday evening and attending the Cornerstone Program five days each week.

I have not received a response from my last letter of January 29, 2007, in which I requested an explanation of the diluted result reported on January 11, 2007 from the specimen you submitted on January 5, 2007.

Please fax or e mail an explanation of this result. As previously noted, you are requested to refrain from consuming liquids two hours prior to a test which may cause a dilute result.

Please contact me if there are any additional questions, or inform me immediately if you choose not to comply with these requests. Your cooperation in these matters is appreciated.

Sincerely,

Bernard Karmatz, M.S., LMFT
Diversion Program Case Manager

cc: file
Sent by fax and mail

Figure 15

I must admit that by now I was getting a bit frustrated with Mr. Karmatz. I sent him a return letter and decided to seek advice from members of the diversion program.

They all had incredible insight ranging from the fact that most thought our friend Bernie (Mr. Karmatz) was simply a prick to those who questioned if I needed to be there in the first place. These people in this program were impressive to me. They all had had a problem that they confronted head on and I respected them for that. They also acknowledged that at the time of their inclusion into the group they needed to be there. Almost all admitted to being a mess when they arrived. And that, according to the consensus of the group, was the basis for my problem with Bernie. I wasn't a mess. I arrived with none of their issues and a clean bill from Hazelden. I didn't have to take Bernie's crap, and I didn't.

But as I said before, the Medical Board of California is a bit more sinister. Due process is not a part of their mantra. Despite my communications all along with Mr. Valine, I received a letter from him with all kinds of innuendo ignoring every conversation and letter I had copied to him. It would seem that the fish that is the Medical Board of California stinks from the head.

In August of 2006 I was contacted by a Ms. Robin Hollis, a Senior investigator, for the Medical Board of California. Doctor-patient privilege presents me from discussing the particulars of the case, but after a telephone conversation she informed me that they would like me to come in and review the case face-to-face with their examiner. I told her I would be happy to do that. I then received a fax detailing what she really meant.

Not once during our conversation did she suggest that she was going to need any of the items in her letter. I felt sideswiped. At the least she had been less than genuine. I told her I would have to speak to my attorney before I could commit to a meeting. I also demonstrated my disdain that this whole thing seemed to be driven by a witch hunt involving another physician.

Jan R. Adams MD

February 26, 2007

Bernard Karmatz MS, LMFT
Diversion Program Case Manager

Dear Mr Karmatz:

I am in receipt of your letter dated February 21, 2007. I must add that I am a bit confused by your request. You offer that " after administrative review", you are requesting that I "begin the outpatient program at the Cornerstone facility this week".

Yet, you are unable to tell me when the administrative review took place, who performed the review and why, and how that decision was made. On two previous occasions you have offered that "Sacramento" had sent down the directive, yet my conversations with Frank Valine proved that those statements by you were less than accurate. In fact, Mr Valine offered that he had had no such conversations.

I am further concerned about your request because I have previously interviewed at Cornerstone with Jan McClary and Bonnie McClain, the Senior Intake Coordinator and Manager, respectively, and they both, in lieu of my report from Hazelden, were at a loss to determine exactly what you thought I required treatment for. I have previously shared this with you in a letter dated the 19th of January 2007.

As for complying with the terms of the Diversion agreement that I signed on December 14, 2006, I am further confused by that statement from you. I have attended every scheduled meeting and taken every random drug test, none of which have been positive. This also was addressed in my letter dated January 29, 2007 and so I having a bit of trouble interpreting your posture as anything but hostile, and I am concerned.

Previously, I asked you what the requirements were to secure a DEC meeting. Your response was "what is DEC?" However in your letter dated January 16, 2007 you offered that I could not be scheduled for a Diversion Evaluation Committee meeting. What was that? I wonder if these words mean anything to you:... "Soon after applying for participation in the Diversion Program, each prospective participant is evaluated by a Diversion Evaluation Committee (DEC). The DEC establishes an individual rehabilitation plan (Diversion Agreement) for each doctor in Diversion"... It seems to me (and a lot of other people involved in the program) that you make it up as you go along and then try to pass on your opinions as directives coming from your superiors.

As for your having "not received a response from your letter dated January 29, 2007" I will refax and attach a copy of my response dated that same day. You try to make the issue of a dilute urine a point of contention, but fail to acknowledge that neither alcohol nor ethyl glucuronide was present. That is after all, the purpose of the test.

Figure 16

Perhaps though, after nearly three months of voluntary participation, its time for me to make a decision if diversion is right for me. I know it has caused problems for you because I do not fit your paradigm: your experts at Hazelden could not pin the diagnosis of alcoholism or alcohol dependency on me, and frankly I think you resent that.

Sincerely

Jan R. Adams MD

cc: Tom Byrne, Esq
Henry Fenton, Esq
Marsha Vanover, Phd
Frank Valine, Director Diversion Program

Figure 16 (continued)

Mar-02-07 03:15P 916 263 2607 P.01

STATE OF CALIFORNIA -- STATE AND CONSUMER SERVICES AGENCY ARNOLD SCHWARZENEGGER, Governor

Consumer Affairs

MEDICAL BOARD OF CALIFORNIA
PHYSICIAN'S DIVERSION PROGRAM
1420 Howe Avenue, Suite 14
Sacramento, CA 95825-3236
Telephone: (916) 263-2600
Toll Free: 1-866-728-9907
www.mbc.ca.gov

March 2, 2007

Jan Rudalgo Adams, M.D.
553 Emerald Bay
Laguna Beach, CA 92651

Dear Dr. Adams:

On December 14, 2006, you signed an Agreement During Evaluation Process with the Medical Board of California's Physician Diversion Program. Number two of this Agreement states, "I will enter a treatment program within one to seven days as directed if it is determined by the Diversion Program that treatment is necessary in order for me to practice medicine safely. The cost will be at my expense."

Since you have not entered the treatment program as directed, you will no longer be allowed to participate in the evaluation phase of the Diversion Program. This decision became effective on February 27, 2007. Since you are no longer eligible to participate, you cannot attend the Diversion Group Meetings. If you decide that you would like to reapply to enter the Diversion Program, you must first enter the treatment program recommended, then contact the Diversion Office in Sacramento to complete a new telephone intake.

Although you are not participating in the Diversion Program, we hope you will continue to pursue recovery.

Sincerely,

Frank L. Valine
Diversion Program Administrator

FLV:rb

cc: Marsha Vanover, Ph.D.
Bernard Karmatz

Figure 17

Jan R. Adams MD

March 2, 2007

Frank Valine
Diversion Program Administrator
Medical Board of California
1420 Howe Avenue, Suite 14
Sacramento, CA 95825

Dear Mr. Valine:

It is quite true that on December 14, 2006, I, Jan R. Adams MD, signed an Agreement During Evaluation Process with the Medical Board of California's Physician Diversion Program. That agreement was also signed by your representative Bernard Karmatz MS, LMFT.

It is also true that Number Two of this Agreement states that " I will enter a treatment program within one to seven days as directed if it is determined by the Diversion Program that treatment is necessary in order for me to practice medicine safely. The cost will be at my expense."

You then go on to suggest that I did "not enter the treatment program as directed".

I submit to you a letter sent to me by Mr. Karmatz dated October 10, 2006. (I'm going to allow that the date submitted by Mr Karmatz is incorrect.) In it, he presents three treatment facilities for me to contact, including Hazelden Springbrook, which I entered in January when a bed became available. Mr Karmatz was privy to this entire process. I was discharged after three days with them confirming that a diagnosis of alcohol dependency could not be made according to the criteria set forth in the DSM IV. In other words , this individual is not an alcoholic.

Literally before I returned home Mr Karmatz was planning for me to enter a treatment facility. The problem was that he didn't have the diagnosis he had counted on, and frankly, the people at Cornerstone, like me, were at a lost to determine exactly what it was that Mr Karmatz thought they should be treating.

I spoke with you about this matter and you, yourself, confirmed that "we were getting ahead of ourselves", and that "we should wait for the report from Hazelden Springbrook" and "take it one day at a time".

Now, I get a letter dated March 2, 2007, from you (and signed by Rhonda) trying to suggest that I had in someway violated the Agreement During Evaluation Process and frankly I am stunned. I truly thought you were a better person than that. I've come to expect that behavior from Mr Karmatz, but this is a bit alarming.

Figure 18

In the last three months since signing the Agreement, I have not missed a meeting and I have not had a positive urine test. I would also suggest that besides Number Two in the Agreement During Evaluation Process, there are Thirteen other provisions and none of these have been violated.

In a conversation with Rhonda today, she inquired that "if I didn't think I had a problem then why am I in diversion anyway?" My answer was simply this: After having sat through a number of meetings I realized that it didn't necessarily have to be about drugs or alcohol: all of us can benefit from taking a look inside ourselves to determine some of the things we need to do in order to be better people. I found that the individuals in diversion have a lot of insight into life, period.

And so, if you believe that diversion may not be the right place for me I will respect that. But I will not allow you, or Mr Karmatz, to fabricate reasons to justify that. Simply say that it isn't a fit. No one need be at fault.

And finally, an issue of even greater importance is the final statement in your letter: "Although you are not participating in the Diversion Program, we hope you will continue to pursue recovery." Your experts at Hazelden Springbrook conceded that, after evaluation, I did not meet the DSM IV criteria for alcohol dependency. Therefore, one would think that an individual charged in life with the task of running a program like Diversion, would recognize that there is nothing from which to recover (except the horrifying experience that there are career bureaucrats out there, like your Mr Karmatz, who would cling to checking a box on a form, regardless of the data; someone who can offer no insight, only labels).

Sincerely:

Jan R. Adams MD

CC: Tom Byrne, Esq
Henry Fenton, Esq
Marsha Vanover Phd
Bernard Karmatz -

Figure 18 (continued)

08/01/2006 15:11 8185512131 MEDICAL BOARD OF CA PAGE 02/03

STATE OF CALIFORNIA – STATE AND CONSUMER SERVICES AGENCY ARNOLD SCHWARZENEGGER, Governor

Consumer Affairs

MEDICAL BOARD OF CALIFORNIA
ENFORCEMENT PROGRAM
OFFICE OF INVESTIGATIVE SERVICES
Valencia District Office
27202 Turnberry Lane, Suite 280
Valencia, CA 91355
Tel. (661) 295-3397 Fax (661) 295-3030
www.caldocinfo.ca.gov

August 1, 2006

Jan Adams, M.D.
1033 Hilgard Avenue, #9
Los Angeles, CA 90024

Dear Dr. Adams:

This is to confirm the interview arrangements made during our telephone conversation today. The interview is scheduled for 11:00 a.m. tomorrow, August 2, 2006, at the Medical Board of California District Office, located at 320 Arden Avenue, Suite 250, Glendale, CA 91203

Please bring a photo identification, your current Curriculum Vitae and any other documents, records or other materials that you believe will be relevant to the discussion. You are welcome to bring an attorney to the interview if you wish, but you are not obligated to do so. This interview will be tape recorded and upon request, a copy of the tape recording will be provided to you at no charge. You may also bring your own tape recording device should you wish to do so. In addition, when the Board has concluded its review, you will be notified of the outcome.

I have enclosed directions to the Glendale District Office. Please contact me at (818) 551-2125 if you are unable to attend the scheduled interview.

Sincerely,

Robin Hollis
Senior Investigator

Enc.

Cc: 17-2006-172927/17-2006-175650

Figure 19

Jan R. Adams MD

1 August, 2006

Robin Hollis
MBC
27202 Turnberry Lane, Suite 280
Valencia CA 91335

Dear Ms. Hollis:

I'm afraid your letter confirms nothing about the arrangements we made during our telephone conversation today. What it does confirm is the dishonesty and the self serving manner in which you conduct business. During our entire conversation you mentioned none of the details you try to put forth as having been discussed in your letter.

My attorney cannot clear his schedule in order to be present tomorrow and expresses dismay that you would suggest he be there with less than 20 hours of warning.

I know that during another physician's hearing the board questioned him on whether I was having money problems. He mentioned that because he was stunned. My situation had absolutely nothing to do with his case and he felt it inappropriate that you people would ask that. I guess you are not bound by the rule of law or the rule of decency.

I will consult with my attorney as to when he might be available.

I will be out of the country on business from August 5 through August 18, 2006. I wqill do my best to accommodate you.

Sincerely

Jan R. Adams MD

Figure 20

The meeting was confirmed for August 3, 2006 in her office. I met with her and her investigator, a physician I did not know. He began by going through the fine print of the chart and this went on for about an hour. When finally my patience had been exhausted, I asked him where this was going.

He put me off, and continued going through the detail of the chart. Ultimately, it came down to this: the recovery room nurse had written that the patient was received in the recovery room at 14:25 hours. The anesthesia record showed that the patient had been discharged from the operating room at 12:25 hours. I was being harassed to explain to the Medical Board of California what had happened in those two hours.

I explained that my review of the chart demonstrated that the patient had no problems. The anesthesia report confirms that the patient was wheeled the twenty feet to the recovery room. The anesthesiologist signed her in to recovery at 12:25. Maybe, just maybe, the nurse couldn't tell time. At any rate what they needed to do was ask the nurse, not me. Needless to say, I made no new friends that day. It's okay though, the Medical Board of California isn't looking for friends. They are looking to justify their own existence.

Now don't get me wrong: I understand the position of the Medical Board of California concerning physicians and substance abuse and I support their efforts. I also believe when you are wrong, you own it, correct it, make amends for it, and then move on with the intention of doing better. I humbly submit to that.

With that in mind I am more than willing to fulfill whatever obligations they deem appropriate. But I will not be forced to own something that is not mine. I will not allow other people to apply labels to me that do not speak to who I am.

I think it's fair to say Mr. Karmatz now understands that whether he accepts it or not. I personally do not require that of him. What I require of him is what I have always required of him and that is while he goes about his job from day to day never forget that at the other end of their policy is a human being.

Further along in his appearance on Larry King Live, Harvey Levin stated that "and the medical board—at least the executive director—doesn't think he should be practicing".

So, I asked them about that statement and this was their reply:

STATE AND CONSUMER SERVICES AGENCY - *Department of Consumer Affairs* Arnold Schwarzenegger, *Governor*

MEDICAL BOARD OF CALIFORNIA
Executive Office

May 20, 2008

Jan R. Adams, M.D.
11819 Wilshire Blvd., Suite 214
Los Angeles, CA 90025

Dear Dr. Adams:

In response to your inquiry of May 19, 2008, this is to confirm that neither I nor the executive director of the Medical Board of California has ever told any member of the media that our board "has been trying to get (your) license for some time."

Sincerely,

Candis Cohen

Candis Cohen
Information Officer

2005 Evergreen Street, Suite 1200, Sacramento, CA 95815-3831 (916) 263-2389 Fax (916) 263-2387 www.mbc.ca.gov

May 20 08 02:36p 3104448809 p.2

Figure 21

In an attempt to draw me out and obtain attention for himself by forcing me into a one-on-one interview with him, Harvey then began to display the particulars of my divorce. Nonetheless, again he only presented half the story. He reported that there had been a restraining order filed against Dr. Adams, and certainly the suggestion was that this guy is somehow mean or violent, both of which are not the case. Again, I find this to be almost blasphemous because if he obtained that data, then he got the whole report and therefore, to present half the story is criminal. Item 27, which refers to personal conduct restraining orders, states very clearly in the first paragraph that both parties shall be subject to personal conduct restraining orders, with both parties restrained and protected from the other party. That seems to be pretty much clear as far as I can tell.

Nonetheless, there was also a letter from my ex-wife's attorney which clearly pointed out that "as of tomorrow, January 29, 2007, I will appear in court and continue and reissue the temporary orders one last time to allow you and Ms. Field time to complete your preliminary declarations of disclosure." Her attorney further goes on to say, "Once the above is completed, I will dismiss the entire domestic violence action as previously discussed."

They then dug up an ex-girlfriend. It is, however, very true that there is nothing so frightening as a woman scorned. I will not go into details because I think that's silly. But I do think it's important to point out once again that Harvey only told half the story: the half that was mean and harmful to me. He didn't report that that same woman wrote in an e-mail that "if you do not come back to me within 24 hours, you will wish you were never born."

Now that's a person who I certainly would want to have a relationship with. The puzzling part for me is trying to understand exactly what her goal was. If in fact she wanted a relationship, then threatening someone with retaliation if they don't participate is clearly not the way to do it.

FL-180

ATTORNEY OR PARTY WITHOUT ATTORNEY (Name, State Bar number, and address):
John R. Schilling
JOHN R. SCHILLING, APC

4675 MacArthur Court, Ste. 590
Newport Beach, CA 92660
TELEPHONE NO.: (949) 833-8833 FAX NO. (Optional): (949) 833-3883
E-MAIL ADDRESS (Optional):
ATTORNEY FOR (Name): SUSAN FIELD

FOR COURT USE ONLY

FILED
SUPERIOR COURT OF CALIFORNIA
COUNTY OF ORANGE
LAMOREAUX JUSTICE CENTER
FEB 21 2007
ALAN SLATER, Clerk of the Court
BY J. SCHWARTZ

SUPERIOR COURT OF CALIFORNIA, COUNTY OF ORANGE
STREET ADDRESS: 341 THE CITY DRIVE
MAILING ADDRESS: P.O. BOX 14170
CITY AND ZIP CODE: ORANGE, CA 92613-1570
BRANCH NAME: JUVENILE JUSTICE CENTER

MARRIAGE OF
PETITIONER: SUSAN FIELD

RESPONDENT: JAN ADAMS

JUDGMENT

[X] **DISSOLUTION** [ ] **LEGAL SEPARATION** [ ] **NULLITY**
[ ] **Status only**
[ ] **Reserving jurisdiction over termination of marital or domestic partnership status**
[ ] **Judgment on reserved issues**
Date marital or domestic partnership status ends: 5/31/07

CASE NUMBER: 06 D 010745

1. [X] This judgment [X] contains personal conduct restraining orders [ ] modifies existing restraining orders. The restraining orders are contained on page(s) 14-15 of the attachment. They expire on *(date):* 12/31/2009

2. This proceeding was heard as follows: [ ] Default or uncontested [X] By declaration under Family Code section 2336 [ ] Contested
   a. Date: FEB 21 2007 Dept.: L69 Room:
   b. Judicial officer *(name):* FREDERICK P. AGUIRRE [ ] Temporary judge
   c. [ ] Petitioner present in court [ ] Attorney present in court *(name):*
   d. [ ] Respondent present in court [ ] Attorney present in court *(name):*
   e. [ ] Claimant present in court *(name):* [ ] Attorney present in court *(name):*
   f. [ ] Other *(specify name):*

3. The court acquired jurisdiction of the respondent on *(date):* 11-30-06
   a. [X] The respondent was served with process.
   b. [ ] The respondent appeared.

THE COURT ORDERS, GOOD CAUSE APPEARING

4. a. [X] Judgment of dissolution is entered. Marital or domestic partnership status is terminated and the parties are restored to the status of single persons
      (1) [X] on *(specify date):* 5/31/07
      (2) [ ] on a date to be determined on noticed motion of either party or on stipulation.
   b. [ ] Judgment of legal separation is entered.
   c. [ ] Judgment of nullity is entered. The parties are declared to be single persons on the ground of *(specify):*

   d. [ ] This judgment will be entered nunc pro tunc as of *(date):*
   e. [ ] Judgment on reserved issues.
   f. The [X] petitioner's [ ] respondent's former name is restored to *(specify):* Susan Field
   g. [ ] Jurisdiction is reserved over all other issues, and all present orders remain in effect except as provided below.
   h. [ ] This judgment contains provisions for child support or family support. Each party must complete and file with the court a *Child Support Case Registry Form* (form FL-191) within 10 days of the date of this judgment. The parents must notify the court of any change in the information submitted within 10 days of the change, by filing an updated form. The *Notice of Rights and Responsibilities—Health Care Costs and Reimbursement Procedures and Information Sheet on Changing a Child Support Order* (form FL-192) is attached.

Page 1 of 2

Form Adopted for Mandatory Use
Judicial Council of California
FL-180 [Rev. January 1, 2007]

JUDGMENT
(Family Law)

Legal Solutions Plus

Family Code, §§ 2024, 2340, 2343, 2346

Figure 22

fulfilled. Each party further understands that noncompliance with those obligations will result in the court setting aside the judgment.

In so doing, the parties acknowledge that said waiver may affect his or her ability to set aside this Stipulation and/or Judgment as provided by law. Having read an agreed to the forgoing regarding waiver of the Final Declaration of Disclosure:

It is hereby stipulated by and between **Susan Field**, Petitioner and **Jan Adams**, Respondent, to each waive the Final Declaration of Disclosure from the other.

27. PERSONAL CONDUCT RESTRAINING ORDERS

A. Both parties shall be subject to personal conduct restraining orders, with both parties restrained and protected from the other party. Respondent is also restrained from Petitioner three (3) minor children, [redacted], [redacted], [redacted], as protected person(s) as follows:

B. Both parties are enjoined from molesting, attacking, striking, stalking, threatening, sexually assaulting, battering, harassing, or telephoning the other party at work, at home, or on any cellular phone, including, but not limited to, annoying telephone calls as described in Penal Code § 653(m), destroying the personal property of, contacting, either directly or indirectly, by mail, e-mail, voicemail, facsimile, or otherwise, coming within one-hundred (100) yards of the other party's home, work, or vehicle, or disturbing the peace of the other party, and/or Petitioner's minor children, pursuant to Family Code §6218(a)-(c), §6320, §6322, and §6340(a).

C. These personal conduct restraining orders against the

Figure 22 (continued)

parties shall expire three (3) years from the date of filing of this Stipulated Judgment, or 12/31/2009, or until further written agreement of the parties or order of the court, whichever shall first occur.

THE ABOVE IS HEREBY STIPULATED:

DATED: January 26, 2007 SUSAN FIELD, PETITIONER

DATED: January 12, 2007 JAN ADAMS, RESPONDENT

APPROVED AS CONFORMING TO THE AGREEMENT OF THE PARTIES:

JOHN R. SCHILLING, APC

DATED: ~~January~~ Feb 12, 2007

John R. Schilling, Esq.
Attorney for Petitioner

DATED: January 12, 2007 JAN ADAMS, In Pro Per

IT IS SO ORDERED:

DATED: FEB 2 1 2007

JUDGE OF THE SUPERIOR COURT

Figure 22 (continued)

Jan-29-2007 16:52 From-J R SCHILLING +949 833 3883 T-962 P.001/001 F-332

JOHN R. SCHILLING
A PROFESSIONAL CORPORATION

JOHN R. SCHILLING
FELLOW, AMERICAN ACADEMY OF MATRIMONIAL LAWYERS
CERTIFIED FAMILY LAW SPECIALIST

4675 MACARTHUR COURT
SUITE 590, TOWER ONE
NEWPORT BEACH, CALIFORNIA 92660

AREA CODE 949
TELEPHONE: 833-8833
FACSIMILE: 833-3883

January 29, 2007

Via Fax
Dr. Jan R. Adams
553 Emerald Bay
Laguna Beach, Ca

RE: Marriage of Field and Adams

Dear Dr. Adams:

Please be advised that tomorrow, January 29, 2007, I will appear in Court and continue and reissue the temporary orders one last time to allow you and Ms. Field time to complete your Preliminary Declarations of Disclosure and enter the judgment with the Court. I had hoped that this would not be necessary, but I can not dismiss the existing matters until the Disclosure statements have been completed and the Judgment entered. Once the above is completed, I will dismiss the entire Domestic Violence action as previously discussed.

Your appearance is not required at tomorrow's hearing. However, please advise how you would like to receive the reissued orders so as to avoid any further inconvenience.

Very truly yours,

John R. Schilling

JRS:cc

cc: Susy Field

Figure 23

Finally, in order to discredit me, Mr. Levin then tried to suggest that malpractice suits filed by patients were related to my performance as a surgeon. It seemed important at the time to imply that the number of malpractice suits filed against me demonstrated a pattern. They do demonstrate a pattern; however, once again, Harvey was so intent on discrediting me that he missed it. These suits do not only represent an abomination perpetrated against me; it is a symbol of the foulness that has contaminated our entire society. Evaluation shows all of them to be without merit.

However, let's look further. A friend of mine, an anesthesiologist, put together a business plan for a surgery center. His argument was: if we can lower the price sufficiently to cover our costs and provide growth, then we can offer these procedures to women who could not otherwise be able to afford it. He came to me and asked me what I thought.

I thought that was a good idea to offer the services at a reduced rate, and I consented to do surgery in their surgery center one day a week. Unfortunately, we were victims of our own success. The one day that I was there to do surgery grew from seeing three to five patients a day to seeing 40. With that kind of volume, the problem really isn't surgery. The problem is meeting the needs of the patients outside of surgery. They begin to feel they are rushed through follow-up, or that they didn't get to spend enough time with the doctor. This in itself led to animosity. Two processes were working here. It may have been a reduced rate for us but it wasn't for the patients. For many, it had taken quite a bit of effort to pull together that money. There was no additional money. That was all they had.

In those instances where the patient (or the doctor) thought a scar could be improved or further refinement might be in order, a problem arose. The patient, though, had no money to cover operating room costs. Their only recourse, in their minds, was to use legal force to compel doctors to do it for nothing. (I will allow also that some people are just underhanded and will always try to get something for nothing. That, however, does not represent malpractice.)

At any given moment, there are 60,000 open medical malpractice cases involving about 700,000 physicians. Furthermore, as noted by Jeff Segal, M.D., the CEO of *Medical Justice News*, "The national practitioner databank includes the names of over 200,000 healthcare professionals who have not only been sued but have paid a settlement or judgment. So, being sued, as noted by Dr. Segal, is hardly an indictment of incompetence, although the media would have you believe otherwise." There's even more incentive if your doctor is the guy on TV (and that would be me).

Also, when these suits occur, you will find that the plaintiff's attorney sues a host of people—the anesthesiologist, the surgery center, and the surgeons—all at once in an effort to divide and conquer and also get the most money for his work. During these procedures, the plaintiff's attorney provides an expert who argues that the treatment in his opinion is below the standard of care. The defense, on the other hand, pays an expert who says, "No, I've reviewed this case and the level of care is not below the standard." I suggest to Mr. Levin that he do his own research and contact the attorneys representing neither the plaintiff nor the defendant but the surgery center. The attorney representing the surgery center in every case I've been associated with has called my attorney and confessed that in spite of all this, their group of experts has never found that Dr. Adams' care was below the standard. Perhaps the problem is that the journalistic time of Woodward and Bernstein, when reporters checked and double-checked their facts, has died a similar death as common decency. Perhaps in their rush to be first, any truth that is reported is purely an accident.

There is, however, one case that deserves a personal comment. There was a patient who had won a judgment due to a sponge having been left in a breast pocket at the time of placement of breast implants. That patient, a Ms. Lori Ufondu, did not come to Dr. Adams; she came to another surgeon who in fact was named as the lead surgeon in her case. I happened to be in this doctor's facility at the time she presented. He asked me to see this patient because she had had surgery previously, and he wanted to get another opinion. I examined her and suggested that he place her implants under the muscle because she was thin, and complaining that she could see wrinkling. Generally, that is the result of an implant that is under filled, but it can occur when there is not enough tissue to adequately camouflage the implant. Placing it below the muscle, though not perfect, would allow him to camouflage it better. He asked that I be present when the surgery occurred because he had never done that surgery before.

Ms. Ufondu apparently had the procedure done and I can't comment on whether I was present as an assistant or the primary surgeon. She did not win her case because she, or her lawyer, demonstrated that one of the doctors was at fault: she won her case because the surgery center had misplaced her chart and was unable to find it.

I myself reviewed over 200 augmentation mammoplasties that I have done. I have used lap pads and never a sponge. I do that because that's exactly what I was taught. The person who taught me breast surgery was Ed Wilkins at the University of Michigan. Ed is a tremendous surgeon who is incredibly meticulous. He never allowed a sponge in the operating room during this procedure because when they're wet, they're like tissue paper. This is a practice that has followed me throughout my career. Since I have never used a sponge in these types of cases, the likelihood after reviewing 200 cases that I did it are minimum. Nonetheless, I believe that surgeons should take responsibility for the care of patients and sometimes that means even when it is not specifically your fault, and I do that.

I would, however, add that California law requires the presence of a registered nurse in the operating room. One of the duties of the registered nurse is to keep an accurate count of sponges. I doubt seriously if any surgeon closed an open wound in a patient where a nurse advised that the sponge count was incorrect. Nonetheless, as I said before, it is the surgeon's ultimate responsibility and for that I am more than happy to take the responsibility for Ms. Ufondu. However, I do stand on my position and I will not alter that. I have never used, or allowed, a sponge like the one apparently found in Ms. Ufondu on the surgical field, in my twenty-year career, period.

4

People attack because of fear. An attack is a call for help.

I FIRST LEARNED that as a resident in surgery. I trained in a program that was brutal. I was on call every other day every other weekend for five years with approximately 60 attending staff members who clearly thought you only worked for them. A typical day would begin at 5:30 a.m. and end the next day at 7:00, or 8:00 p.m. That's right, the next day at 8:00 p.m. You literally were at the hospital for 38 to 40 hours straight.

Nevertheless, there was always a lull at around 2:00 or 3:00 a.m. when you could rest. Invariably though, that is when the night nurse would call with some ridiculous question. You learned very early in your career to hate her. She knew you had been there all day. She knew you were absolutely exhausted. The question then, was always: why is she calling me at this moment, right when I can close my eyes for a second?

The answer was simple: she called because she needed help.

What happened next challenged me to my core. It was easy for me to shrug off the press because I knew they were all wrong. It, however, was not easy to sit back and watch the people I loved being hurt by what the press was saying. And what they were saying was mean. I say that because the press knew they were operating in a climate where, as a doctor, you couldn't defend yourself. They all knew that any discussion of the facts would ultimately lead to a discussion of Donda West, but they didn't care. My service was receiving a hundred calls an hour, and the mailbox on my cell was filling up faster than I could answer it. I finally resolved that the only thing to do was shut it off and let the process run its course.

The problem was it refused to burn out. I finally posed the question to Amy Keith of *People Magazine*: If it's against the law for the doctor to violate doctor-patient privilege, isn't it against the law for a reporter to ask him to do that? Is not asking a doctor to break a law conspiracy to commit a crime? She simply shrugged and offered that she had to try.

Larry King, to his credit, got it. The fiasco had started on his show, but he clearly understood there was a lot more to the story. He also correctly understood that, ultimately, the only one who could make it right was me.

I, however, first needed the coroner to clear me, which he did.

Two questions still remain: why did the press take this posture in the first place, and secondly, why did the so-called legitimate news people join in?

It would be easy to blame tabloid news organizations for getting this off on the wrong foot but that would be unfair. Harvey Levin, for all his bravado, is really just a pawn in all this. There are those who think Mr. Levin is a bad person. I don't share their sentiment. A person or a thing is not intrinsically good or bad. Goodness or badness is merely a subjective value judgment that we assign to a person or event to indicate whether we agree with them or not. (The joke amongst my friends is that I must have dated Harvey's sister. That's the only way to explain the tenacity of his venom.)

I believe Harvey and TMZ were being used. I believe that the person responsible for her aftercare realized early on that he was negligent in her care and that, in order to remain close to the source of money in his family, he had better point the finger elsewhere.

I believe the plan to do that was orchestrated with the help of entertainment lawyers. And I believe the inaccurate information shared by Harvey Levin on "Larry King Live" was coming from that camp.

Now don't get me wrong Harvey and TMZ have to take responsibility for their part. They began a malicious assault by contacting my patients. They called a patient who had a breast lift and tummy tuck two years earlier. They placed post-operative photos of her on their site with the caption, "the butchery of Dr. Adams". They engaged in defamation when they misled the public by posting pictures taken one week after surgery, the day the drains were removed. They engaged in defamation when they omitted the fact that she was scheduled one month later for a procedure. They committed defamation when they told her that nobody's going to want to do surgery with him when we are done. They committed defamation when they encouraged her to cancel her procedure.

Yet what was the press to think when next, a Dr. Aboolian appeared on television offering that he had seen Dr. West in consultation. On camera, sitting at a desk with a chart in front of him, he began going through her history and physical. If I were a member of the media and knew nothing of doctor-patient privilege, I would certainly think, "What does Dr. Adams have to hide?" He's telling us a Code of Ethics prevents him from discussing a patient, but it doesn't seem to hinder this guy. Furthermore the California Medical Board, the American Board of Plastic Surgery, and more importantly, the family and their lawyers weren't demanding that Aboolian cease and desist. Clearly his behavior violates every tenet of doctor-patient privilege.

What was even more astounding, however, was that Dr. Aboolian first suggested that the patient had heart disease and that is why he wouldn't do surgery, and then retracted to say she would not get evaluated and that is why he would not operate. Neither statement is true. We both know (or at least should have known) Ms. West's cardiac status had already been evaluated and cleared a few months earlier at Cedars-Sinai Medical Center, as noted by the coroner.

Dr. Phil McGraw, whose apparent arrogance knows no limits, went even further. He put on a show in which three former patients of mine told their story. Phil stepped way over the line in a number of ways. Number one, he produced an envelope suggesting that he had gotten clearance from these patients in order for me to be present on his show. Nonetheless, my attorney had requested copies of the so-called releases on a number of occasions and had still yet to receive them.

Number two, Dr. Phil stated that I had consented to come on his show, but nothing was further from the truth. I had told Dr. Phil McGraw and his assistant that I was not doing any shows at this time, and that, at the very least, it was inappropriate for me to do them. I did offer a concession. I told him that in the future when it's appropriate for me to do so, and if the appropriate releases are obtained, then I would be more than willing at some time to come on his show and discuss it.

But Phil is a bully. Initially his posture was to be soft and accommodating, to embrace me as a colleague. He offered that he had evaluated many patients psychologically for surgery in the past and knew what I was going through. He wanted his show to be balanced. He had seen these types of patients in the past in his own practice. Yet when I declined to attend, his posture quickly changed to anger and he made it clear the show was going to go on without me. I have done over 4,000 surgical procedures, my last point to Phil was, if he wanted his show to be balanced, allow those 3,997 other people to sit in the audience while these three presented their case.

But apparently that is not Dr. Phil at all. We now know that Dr. Phil has gone unsolicited to a hospital to see a patient: a hospital where he is not on staff in a state where he is not licensed.

We also know that he arranged bail for criminals in order to get an exclusive.

I would also offer that it was this kind of malicious defamation on the part of cattleman that he himself is now spinning toward me that brought him and Oprah together in the first place.

At any rate, Ms. Ufondu who was on his show has already been discussed. Hypertrophic scarring in a woman of color is nowhere near malpractice or below the standard of care. It has to do with how people heal. The third patient, a LPN, still owes our office $5,000 and her presence there was to create an air of defensiveness on our part. She simply is trying to avoid paying the remainder of her bill.

So that's how it all got started, but there is one more factor that contributed to why the press chose to run with it. Remember, at the onset, I pointed out that "people attack because of fear. An attack is a call for help." So what does the press fear? What help do they need?

They fear extinction. They need a way to survive.

The fact is the influence of large media companies is dying. The internet and the notion of social media have changed the business model. The superficial coverage of a few "big" stories is not enough. Smaller networks of people who are passionate about an issue can now engage in a "conversation" online, often in real time. Marketers have shifted some of their dollars to the net and this trend will only increase. That spells death for newspapers, magazines, and some video journalists. That is why they swarm around a story. That is why they engage in a feeding frenzy without checking the facts. Tomorrow there may be nothing to eat. Citizen journalists will have taken their plate.

Therefore if the media wants to protect its 'food supply' they simply have to join the conversation. The majority won't make it because of arrogance. The one startling thing I learned about a great number of journalists during this ordeal was that they don't listen. I watched horrified while one after the other ignored the facts of the case surrounding Dr. West's death. I cringed in disbelief as they continued to print articles about her so-called heart disease despite the coroner's report to the contrary. They had an angle to their story, most likely suggested by their editor, and no amount of facts was going to change that.

Perhaps it is better that they don't survive. The notion that a few individuals should filter the information we all consume is ludicrous. Bring on the citizen journalist.

5

A FAIR QUESTION THOUGH IS, WHO AM I? I WAS BORN RUDALGO Alonzo Adams in Middletown, Ohio, on April 21, 1954. My parents, Charles Adams and Gwendolyn Roberts, had been married approximately one year earlier at the ripe old age of 18. My father was in the Navy and stationed in Panama and very early my mother moved there to be with him. And so my early years as Rudalgo Alonzo Adams were spent in Central America in the Canal Zone. I don't really have much of a recollection of that time. The first memory I truly have of Panama is actually leaving. There is an image of a very large ship and me looking overboard and thinking, "My God, the water is a long way down."

My first recollection of Middletown, Ohio, where I grew up really begins at about four years of age. By that time, my parents had separated. I have an infant baby sister, and I am living on Sycamore Street with my grandmother and my mother's younger siblings, all in their teens. The house on Sycamore Street was a large, red brick building. It was an odd-shaped house and that made for lots of places for a kid to play, to hide, and to think on his own. By now, my name had been changed by my mother from Rudalgo Alonzo Adams to Jan Rudalgo Adams. Rudalgo Alonzo was way too ethnic.

There were no white kids growing up in our area of Sycamore. In fact, Middletown was quite segregated. The greatest advantage in growing up in Middletown, however, was that you felt safe. Me and the other children who grew up on Sycamore would spend hours playing football in the field across the street during the fall, and baseball in that same field during the summer. What I remember most is just being able to run—free to run.

My greatest Christmas as a child was the year I got my first Chuck Taylor Converse All-Star basketball shoes. It was a signal that I was growing up. I had changed from the nondescript 99¢ sneakers to a real shoe with a name. That Christmas there was a light snow but even that couldn't hold me back. I bundled myself up, put on my new sneakers, and went outside to run. I had to break them in.

My grandmother, Alice Roberts, was a beautiful and kind woman and what was particularly interesting was that she, along with my grandmother Alberta about 12 miles away in Hamilton, Ohio, were the people who really raised me. When you think about it, 18-year-olds, though having the ability to reproduce children, don't have the ability to rear them. They are still trying to discover who they are. In America we consider this as dysfunctional, being away from your birth parents most of the time, but I believe that grandparents are in fact more able to take on that task. They are more patient, they certainly have the wisdom of time, and more importantly, they are not trying to discover who they are. They are really trying to share with you who you can be.

That is why the most devastating moment in my life still rings true as if it happened yesterday. When I was nine, my grandmother Alice Roberts died of a stroke on the living room sofa. I vividly remember the paramedics trying to revive her. I can still see her mouth twisting toward the right side of her face and her eyes rolling back in her head.

Yet the person most affected at that time was my mother. My nickname was Trick and I remember her coming to me crying, holding me and saying, "Trickie, what are we going to do without Grandma?"

I had really no emotion. I didn't know what was going on, or how to feel. I really didn't quite understand that Grandma would in fact be gone. I guess at some level I understood that she would always be with me.

The time after my Grandma's death was lonely for me. I spent more time alone, and books became my companions. I'd sit in a hidden corner in that old house and allow my imagination to run wild.

It was also at that time that I began to psychologically become two different people. Perhaps it is symbolic of my name change. On the one hand, I was that fun, sweet, loving child who spent time with his grandmother, and yet, after her death I became isolated (and extremely protective of the child in me). And so, in a sense, there was Jan, the sweet little kid, and Jan the protector, the strong, wise, defender who would protect that young boy at all costs.

It is also at about this time that I began spending more time with my paternal grandmother, Alberta Hicks. I spent all of my summers with her. She had remarried and had three children—Tony, Patricia, and Paula—who were all much older than me. I don't really remember a lot of time with them. It was basically my time with Grandma and frankly, they were excluded.

My grandmother was really my confidant and my teacher. My mornings would start with her at the kitchen table eating fried potato pancakes and collard greens. That by far was my favorite meal and I would have eaten that three times a day without any complaints if she would have let me.

After breakfast my Grandma and I walked the half block down the street to the Rib Shack, a combination dry cleaner and convenience store my grandparents owned. My grandmother pressed clothes on the dry cleaners side of the store. I wasn't allowed over there. She didn't want me near the steam presses.

My job was to run the convenience store, which consisted of counting change and eating as much candy as I could before lunch time.

Our most tender moment occurred approximately 15 years later. My grandmother was getting older and I was now off to college. I had come home for summer break. (During those times, I always made two trips. The first was to Woodside Cemetery to see my maternal grandmother, Alice Gates Roberts, and tell her how I was doing. I'd wind through the roads of Woodside Cemetery and park all alone in front of her grave, and just get out and talk. It was a peaceful time for me, and it helped me get a lot of things out that I needed to get out. I would then get into the car and continue south to Hamilton, Ohio, and see Alberta.) On this occasion, she was in a very talkative mood and explained to me how she had grown up in Bethel, Ohio, a member of the only black family in town. By now Grandma was in her nineties. Her most vivid remembrance was that of graduation from high school. None of the white kids would walk across the stage to receive diplomas with her. Finally a Jewish girl consented to do it. This Jewish girl, of course, was from the only Jewish family in Bethel. What was interesting to hear was that at 18 years of age, all my grandmother wanted to do was move away from Bethel. She didn't talk of a career. She didn't speak of wanting a family. She just wanted to get away from Bethel, and she did.

She moved to Cincinnati, Ohio, and that's where she met my grandfather, Edward Adams, who had come north from Alabama. I never met Edward Adams and no one ever really talked about him. By the time I was born, Edward had died and my grandmother had remarried Pearlman Hicks, the only Grandpa I knew. Yet here she was, one of the most wonderful people I had ever known, telling me how racism in America had affected her choices, and ultimately, her decision to leave home. That has always stuck with me. It's amazing that people could be so mean to someone who truly was such a wonderful spirit.

At that time I also began to think philosophically about who we all were. It seemed inherent to me that we, as people, were all part of a whole. We are one. And it seemed to me that it was obvious that if we were to survive, we would have to do that together.

But we had yet to evolve. That obvious truth that I could see as a child wasn't so obvious to a lot of grownups.

My parents had divorced by the time I was five and so sports became my father and my teacher after the death of Alice. As a child, I guess you could say I was parentified. My mother was a single parent raising two children on her own. As the oldest, my responsibility was for my younger sister. My mother would leave for work each morning at approximately 6:30 a.m. and from that time forward I was to be responsible for Delia (to this day my best friend).

The hours after school were spent first making sure my sister got home safely? It was then off to whatever sport the season dictated. I played baseball during the summer and was very fortunate because the kid who lived two doors down was John Holland.

John was a tremendous athlete. He eventually played football for the Minnesota Vikings. He and I would go to McKinley Junior High School across the street from our houses with a tennis ball and a baseball bat. We played strikeout almost every day during the spring. It was John Holland who taught me to hit a baseball.

During the fall I played Pee Wee Football. Everyday after school, I would come home, get my bicycle, and pedal the five miles south to Smith Park. I never really thought about it at the time: that the other boys were always there with their fathers and I wasn't; I really didn't think about it. All I really wanted to do was play. It was my time to have fun. I was good at it, and my coaches took an interest in me. It was also the only time that I interacted with white kids in Middletown, except for school.

I didn't see my coaches as the white men from the other side of the town, though; I saw them as uncles and brothers and father figures who had taken an interest in me. Football turned out to be very, very kind to me. It afforded me the attention that all kids need, and soon football would be my ticket out of Middletown.

In grade school and junior high I played on the basketball team, but not after my sophomore year in high school. It was the age of specialization and prudence dictated that I concentrate on football. Fortunately for me, it was a small community and I was the quarterback on the football team.

When I entered high school, my mother became increasingly concerned and a lot more overbearing concerning my development. She saw it as a time when young boys grow wild. She saw it as a turning point: you choose a path that is honorable, or one that leads to destruction. She was taking no chances.

An uncle was the pastor of Mt. Zion Baptist Church. My mother suggested that it might be very good for me, if I became a junior deacon and spent more time around him at this point in my life. I did.

The church though was a strange place for me at thirteen. I understood faith but I guess I just couldn't understand the logic behind it. By this time, books were everything for me, and I was learning to have a lot more questions than people could supply answers. I just remember thinking that my uncle, the Rev. Hampton, wasn't so much interested in saving my soul, as he was in making me a good Baptist.

At any rate, I was on my way to high school, and in Middletown that meant getting on a bus and going from the "hood", to where the white kids lived. I was a sophomore heading to Middletown High School and for me that ultimately meant football. Coach Jack Gordon was destined to be the person who became my father figure.

Even as a sophomore, it was apparent that I was going to be the Middletown Middies quarterback someday. I cherished that. It made me the most popular kid in the sophomore class. It also got me elected president of the sophomore class and placed on the student council.

I had developed my closest friendships by the time I was in high school. Rick Martin and Guy Mack had been friends of mine since grade school. I played football, and Rick and Guy were starting guards on the basketball team. They would come to football games to support me, and in turn, when basketball season arrived I cheered them on. The three of us did everything together. Most of all, we participated in high school life.

In the middle of our sophomore year, Middletown's racism reared its ugly head. During football season, it was traditional for us to select homecoming queen candidates. The problem was that in a school where there were 700 kids in a class and only 100 of them black, the black girls never had an opportunity to participate. That is where the rifts began, and by the time Black History month had arrived, Middletown High School had become separated along racial lines.

As president of the sophomore class, I was required to meet with the student council to discuss these issues. Unfortunately for us, before these meetings could be secured, violence broke out and for a week Middletown High School was closed. The communities separated from each other and, as was traditional, the ministers in the black churches emerged as leaders.

From my perspective though, that was the problem. Slavery and the racism that followed was not a moral issue that required the expertise of ministers. No, slavery at its onset was an economic issue. America with all its land needed free labor to work it. Resolving the race issue therefore needed to start with recognizing the economic contributions that we, as black people, had made to America.

I just couldn't see being angry at a white kid who was just plain ignorant. For one, I didn't see it as his fault. He had been miseducated. He didn't know that a black man invented the third rail, or the traffic light, or the machine that made his shoes. He didn't know that a black man developed the technique for storing blood for transfusions. He didn't know that a black woman invented the washing machine. He hadn't been taught this. As far as he knew all black folks did was take. America made him that way.

The Ku Klux Klan, which everybody believes to be a Southern phenomenon, was actually quite active in our area. Periodically, during the time surrounding the riots at Middletown High, we would get calls to our house that were threatening. That was the most amazing situation for a sixteen year old. I was not particularly militant; in fact, my only dream was to complete high school and get on to college. The Klan, however, saw it differently.

Psychologically, I closed down then, and even though I didn't know it, that was to color how I related to the outside world from then on. I was friendly, I was cordial, but it was clear that I was never going to allow people inside again. To be 16 years old and have the Ku Klux Klan calling your house threatening your life and your family's life was just too much.

Perhaps my personality and my talents were more suited to public office, having been president of the sophomore class, the junior class, and then finally of the student body, but that episode changed me. That's why I chose medicine rather than business or law, and even within medicine I was determined to do research to further minimize my interactions with people.

I applied to Harvard College and was accepted. The summer before I left for school, I worked at Armco Steel Corporation as a general laborer. My job was hysterical. I worked at Project 600.

Project 600 is where the steel is rolled into coils for transport. There were four large furnaces that could achieve temperatures of greater than 2000°F. Raw steel was placed in these furnaces and heated to almost a 'gel' so that it could be molded into different shapes. These furnaces had movable parts that would slide the steel out onto a conveyor to be rolled into coils. These movable parts had to be lubricated with oil, but understandably, it was so hot, that when oil was placed on them, the oil would heat up and liquefy to a point of where it would drip. Approximately 65 feet underground, in the basement, were the working mechanisms of these furnaces.

Now, here we are in Ohio, in the middle of July. It's 95° outside with 95% humidity. I'm 65 feet underground, under furnaces where the temperature is greater than 2000°F, and I have a steam gun removing oil from the floor and forcing it into trenches to be carried away and processed. Needless to say, that job motivated me to study at Harvard.

But Middletown is a good place. When it became apparent that I was on my way to Harvard, the entire town rallied around it.

Even the whites who worked at Armco Steel Corporation were supportive. They too believed that if I did my best at Harvard, with emphasis on the best, I would have the opportunity to enjoy "how the other half lives." It also afforded me an opportunity to come out from under those furnaces periodically to enjoy their air conditioned offices.

6

My mom and I packed three large bags, placing in them the things I would need for college. This included winter clothes and my white football cleats. We struggled with those bags as we placed them in the car and headed for Dayton Airport. When I arrived in Boston I struggled with those bags as I pulled them to the curb. I hailed a taxi, the driver helped me put them in the trunk, and off we went to Harvard Square.

Boston looked old to me. The streets were so narrow and rickety. Yet I knew this was a new beginning. I looked forward to exploring all the history that Boston had to offer. "For goodness sakes, I was on my way to Harvard College," I thought, "the oldest and most prestigious university in America."

The taxi pulled up in front of Hurlbut Hall and let me out. I pulled the luggage to the sidewalk, paid the driver. As he drove off, I stood there looking around. There was a gentle breeze, the trees were green, and the sun was shining brightly. I just stood there. These were the Union dorms which sat outside of Harvard Yard. I pulled my luggage to the front of the building and stared at the doorway. Above the door was a sign that said Hurlbut. The taxi driver had been correct and he had dropped me exactly where I needed to be.

The problem was I had no idea what I needed to do. I stood in front of the door a few moments longer and just looked around. I opened the door to Hurlbut Hall and in the foyer were mailboxes and another door that was locked. On the door was a sign suggesting I go to the next building and meet the janitor. He would give me my keys.

"This is crazy," I thought. "There's no one here to greet us, there's no one here to tell us what to do." I walked to the next building and got the keys from a janitor dressed in blue khakis. "Hurlbut 45," he said, and away I went.

There was no elevator in Hurlbut Hall. I carried those bags up three flights of stairs. I was the second to arrive and my roommate, Ray Swaggerty, had already claimed a bed. I was left with the bed in the front room. Ray was not there and I began to unpack.

My schedule was inside the packet I received from the janitor. Everything that I would need to do for the next few days in order to register was right there.

When I look back on that time, I must have been a sight. Ray Swag finally came in at around 5:00 p.m. We said our hellos but you could see him staring at me: jeans too tight, hair too big, and rose-colored glasses, prescription of course, wire rims certainly. There I was in all my glory.

Ray and I spent a lot of time talking that night. He was from Detroit, he was black, and he was to be my roommate for the next year.

My first task the next day was to find the football stadium. Ralph Goldston, the black coach on the staff, had come to my house in Middletown, Ohio. He was my contact at Harvard. I went across the Charles River to the stadium and registered for football. I was directed to where I needed to go for a physical exam.

Listening to my heart, the doctor immediately noted the irregular heartbeat. I explained that I had just had a physical. I had been nominated to the Naval Academy and they had discovered that I had a Wenckebach heart block. He was uncomfortable with that information. My chart was kicked upstairs. The decision was that I would not play football. I was devastated. The rug had literally been pulled from under my feet. I was lost. I spent the next few days just wandering around Harvard Square.

With each day, though, I became more determined to play. I returned to the doctor and requested a specialist. After a number of examinations, he consented to let me play, and so approximately four weeks late, I joined the freshman football team.

Unfortunately for me, people had already secured positions. I started at the back of the quarterbacks and moved up quickly, but it became apparent that I was not going to move up to the starting job. It had nothing to do with ability, nor did it have anything to do with the coach's willingness to let me play. I just think he believed he was protecting me.

The joy that I had known since I was six years old, the joy I had as a football player, was now gone.

At the end of the season, I joined the freshman basketball team. Personally I wasn't particularly good; I hadn't really played in high school, but I was certainly a good enough athlete to make that team. I played the whole year as a swingman.

Ray and I continued to get closer as friends and to do those things that college kids do. What was hilarious was how hard we worked at trying to do nothing. I was pre-med and Ray was studying business. At the start of the second semester Ray came running into the room excited. "Jan," he said, "I've got the course for us: Statistics. They're actually doing multiplication." Thinking that we had found the ultimate "gut" course, we both signed up for statistics that semester. The course began with combinations and permutations and in fact Ray was correct, it was a gut (to start with). But then the course advanced into chi square and other analysis. I remember laughing hysterically as we were both completely lost. We made it through that course, but so much for guts and so much for listening to Ray Swag. From then on, we decided it was just better that we study the courses we needed to graduate.

It was at that time that I met S. Alan Counter, Ph.D. He was the young black biology professor from the South. He was truly a mentor for us all. He was good looking, he was smart, and his wife was absolutely beautiful.

Dr. Counter took me under his wing and it was from him that I became interested in neurobiology. By that time, I had decided to major in psychology with an emphasis on neurobiological systems. My first research project was with him studying the hearing systems in katydids and crickets. Don't laugh—they're very interesting.

Crickets have large front legs and their hearing systems are actually in their knees. They make noise by rubbing the feathers together on their back. What we studied was lateral inhibition. If you've ever heard yourself on a tape recorder, the one thing that you notice is that it doesn't really sound like you. Your hearing system blocks out your own voice when you talk so that you don't directly stimulate yourself. We were studying how much noise the crickets were making as compared to how much they heard. That was a good time for me. I felt connected to him and it helped me psychologically to move on, to move away from football and more into studying medicine.

Ray and I made friends with Ernie Carter and Barry Lee, both of whom were pre-med. We decided to set up a rooming group together, but that was our second disappointment. Harvard was incorporating Radcliffe into the system and it meant that a number of us would have to live at the Radcliffe dorms rather than Harvard. It was unfortunate because, I, as the first name listed, was considered an athlete. That was one of the factors considered in moving people to Radcliffe. Besides, none of us were legacies, and the houses like Elliot, Leverett or Adams were not in our future.

Those years at Harvard were a time of a tremendous development for me. I went from a small town hick who really didn't know that much about the world to learning about kids from places like Washington DC, New York City, and San Francisco, California. Each of us brought our own U.S. culture to the Harvard experience. The first snow in Boston, as a sophomore, brought out the freshmen from Southern California. They were wearing shorts to enjoy the snow. We considered them crazy and they never served to disappoint us.

The first true white friend I made at Harvard was George Vaughn. George was from San Antonio, Texas. George and I spent a lot of time getting to know each other and challenging our prejudices. George's family owned lumber yards in Texas. They were also part owners of the San Antonio Spurs. George gave me the greatest compliment that anyone could give. A friend of his from South Dakota was also at Harvard. He had to write a paper on race relations. George suggested that he sit down with me. I thought that was fantastic. He believed enough in me, and cared enough about who I was as a person to suggest that I might be able to offer some insight.

During the time that I did research with Dr. Counter, I also took a leave of absence for six months to really decide what I wanted to do. I certainly wanted to go to medical school, but my interaction with him really opened my eyes to solving problems. There was a real consideration on my part to pursue a Ph.D. in biology. I opted for medicine. I was concerned that I had begun to isolate myself too much. Even though I thought I had been hurt enough by life and people, I still desperately needed them. The only choice for me ultimately was medical school. The only choice for medical school was Ohio State University College of Medicine. I had interviewed at Cincinnati and at Case Western Reserve, but the one turnoff for me was how important the interviewers at these institutions thought they were. My attitude was, "Dude, I'm about to graduate from Harvard and trust me, no matter how you slice it, either one of you academically will be a step down." At least Ohio State was happy that I considered them. More importantly, I was happy to be going home.

7

I WAS VERY EXCITED ABOUT GOING TO MEDICAL SCHOOL AT OHIO State. Everyone I had interviewed with there had been very nice to me. I was particularly charmed by a plastic surgeon, Dr. Robert Ruberg. He asked the right questions about where I wanted to be. He demonstrated that if I made the choice of Ohio State, he would certainly be there to help.

Ohio State took in a large number of medical students. There were about 160 my year. Of that, approximately 30 of us went into the independent study program. I chose the independent study program because it just seemed to be civilized. I couldn't see me wasting time in lecture discussion classes having my mind roam as I sat there for hours. Independent study was much more suited to me. I could sit down with a very good book in a very quiet place and get it done.

Here's how the independent study program worked. The course workload was divided into modules. Modules were comprised of the material that needed to be learned in that particular subject. You progressed through the module at your own speed. When you had completed a module, you took an exam. If you passed the exam, you progressed to the next module. If you didn't, then you had to see the professor who wrote it. And frankly, that was something you never ever wanted to do.

The independent study program was run by Dr. Michael Altman, but the real backbones of the program were two women, Dee Eskin and Jodi Skinner. Dee was strictly business and expected of you, your best. She made sure that it got done. Jodi was simply all of our fantasy. They were the administrators with whom you interacted. The goal became to impress Jodi by passing all your tests. If you failed, she'd have to tell you those horrible words, "You need to see the professor."

The people in the independent study program were in fact pretty independent themselves. Most were incredibly smart. Many already had advanced degrees. There were a couple of dentists, a pharmacist, and two engineers. Most were older, some of them married, and so it just worked for their lives based on where they were at the time.

My favorite subject was anatomy, and two of my favorite people were our anatomy instructors, both women. The part of anatomy that intrigued me most was embryology. Getting a look at how we develop amazed me. That anybody—and I mean anybody—was born normal was the exception. There were so many things that could go wrong all along the way.

About two months before I was to complete the independent study program and head for the clinical wards at Ohio State Hospitals, I began to feel ill. I experienced a lot of chest pain and after I had had a number of episodes, I decided to talk to one of my instructors about it.

Of course, I went straight to one of my anatomy professors, and was referred to a cardiologist, Dr. Donald Unverferth. It was particularly interesting to meet him because our backgrounds were similar, though his was clearly more impressive than mine.

Donald Unverferth had grown up in Dayton, Ohio near Middletown. He had played football at Ohio State, and had even played quarterback during some of the glory years. He had been drafted by Vince Lombardi of the Green Bay Packers and chose not to go into the NFL. He chose to be a doctor. He was impressive. He was 6'4" tall, still about 210 pounds, prematurely gray hair but still looking young, and all the secretaries and all the nurses loved him.

Donald ordered a lot of tests to examine my heart. It was all very confusing for me. Then one day he came to me looking more serious than usual. We sat down, and he began to talk about what he thought was going on. His concern was not only the Wenckebach block, but that I had developed a cardiomyopathy. My heart was getting larger and larger over time, becoming a more ineffective pump, and the heart rhythms were now becoming increasingly erratic.

I became incredibly sad and even angry following that conversation. Why was this happening to me? I'm the athlete here. I'm the one running every day. I'm the one lifting weights. I'm the one trying to eat right. And yet here I am, 26 years old, and essentially dying of heart disease.

Dr. Unverferth decided to place me in the hospital to run more tests. The first was an electrophysiology study, a very interesting test to undergo. You are completely awake. Electrodes are placed in your groin and in your right arm and pushed into your heart. Different medicines are infused to stimulate your heart and the electrodes record the different rhythms.

The cardiologists discovered that I had an ectopic focus of tissue near my sinoatrial node and that this was most likely the reason for the Wenckebach block. The cardiomyopathy was viral in nature, and an echovirus was cultured. I spent the next 42 days in the cardiac intensive care unit while the cardiologist figured out what medicines would make my heart a more effective pump. At the end of those 42 days, I was on Hydralazine, a vasodilator, Digoxin to help the pump, and Inderal to slow down my heart rate. Oddly enough, one of the side effects of Inderal was to make me confused and it became more difficult to study. As a result I took some time off from school.

A short time later, I began to experience problems with my right knee and subsequently saw another Unverferth, Donald's brother. He was an orthopedic surgeon. It was funny to watch them joke with each other. They sort of used me as a ball to play with. Donald always suggested that I never go into surgery because I wasn't quite dumb enough. His brother would always laugh and say that's exactly why I should go into surgery, because I'm not quite dumb enough to be an internist. They loved each other and it was wonderful to see.

The saddest conversation I've ever had with my mother came after her conversation with Dr. Unverferth. His fear was that this heart disease was progressive. He thought I'd be lucky to get to 44 years of age. Sadly, Dr. Unverferth himself, who was born on exactly the same day as I was although more than a few years earlier, died a couple of years later at the age of 44. He had developed a brain tumor. On the day I received that news, I simply cried.

A few months after being discharged from the CCU, I returned to the wards on the cardiology service. As luck would have it, my first patient was a 42-year-old football coach from a small town in Ohio who had developed a cardiomyopathy. Over the next 30 days, I took care of him. I saw him every day. I watched this vibrant young man take on approximately 200 pounds of water and drown in his own body fluids. That was the reason for Dr. Unverferth's concern for me. Most people with a viral cardiomyopathy don't survive. In a sense, I became the poster child for people with that disease. Before Dr. Unverferth died, periodically, he would come around the ward, collect me, and take me back to the cardiac intensive care unit. He was determined to show his patients that you could survive that disease.

I just enjoyed being with him.

I took to surgery immediately. The chairman of the department at OSU was Larry Carey, and he was a tough bastard whom I loved. He seemed always to be looking at me. No matter how tough he was being, he would give me that smile that kind of said, "You get it? There is no room for error here."

I was interested in neurosurgery at the time, and in my next rotation spent a lot of time with the neurosurgical residents. They were all extremely nerdy, but they were a great group of guys who loved what they were doing. They spent pretty much all their time at the hospital. I talked seriously with Dr. Hunt, who was the chairman of neurosurgery, while on that rotation. He candidly told me that he thought I was a whole lot more like Larry Carey than I was like Bill Hunt. That's when I learned a big lesson. Awareness is the most important thing in life. A lot of times we walk through our days in a fog. We don't really think about what it is that we do. We do it and think about it later. What Bill Hunt had shown me was that it's important to take a look at yourself, be honest with yourself, know who you are, and make an informed decision about who you want to be.

I also learned that we do very harmful things to each other. By continually trying to tie someone to their past, we do them a disfavor. The past is not where we are and it's not where we live. The past is gone. Human beings try to tie each other to the past, but God wants you always to look to the future. The future is where your truth lies. The future is where your life lies.

I chose Lenox Hill Hospital in New York City for general surgery residency. The interview sold me completely. I met Felicien Steichen, who was chairman of the department of surgery at Lenox Hill Hospital, the New York Medical College affiliate at the time and later the Cornell University affiliate and that was all it took. There were a number of things that I liked about Lenox Hill Hospital, but the most important was, its residency program paid the highest salary in the country. I also liked the fact that all the big time Park Avenue surgeons brought their patients there. I knew I wanted to learn surgery from the best, and the old German hospital had a list of the best surgeons in New York City.

Lenox Hill Hospital, as I have mentioned earlier, had a pyramid program, and that was the most frightening part about it. You had approximately 60 masters, because there were 60 general surgeons on staff, and you knew every second of every day one of them was watching you. You had to perform every moment of every day, or fear alienating one of those surgeons who could vote against you returning. The problem was, if you didn't return, you had a hard time finding a place somewhere else. Each of those programs had already taken in the general surgery residents they expected to matriculate through the system. New guys weren't being brought in to be chief resident.

I was closest to Dr. Doug Heyman. Most of the interns and residents were afraid of him. In a sense, he was intimidating, but it was really his desire to make certain that the treatment of his patients was perfect that drove him. There was no, absolutely no, margin for error. And so I did exactly what Dr. Heyman expected of me and I believe it was him who championed my matriculation through the system.

Of particular fun for me was the fact that he had a young daughter, Alexa, who in a sense gave me back some humanity. Lenox Hill Hospital's general surgery program required you to be on call every other night and every other weekend. There wasn't a lot of personal time. On Saturdays, your day off, you'd meet the attendings at the hospital and go on rounds.

Dr. Heyman used Saturday to spend with his daughter and there were times when he would bring her to the hospital with the intention of spending the remainder of day with her. If he got tied up, this six-year-old and I would have lunch.

I attended her Bat Mitzvah. It was both joyous and sad. I listened as my little friend recited the scriptures she was required to memorize. Her words made me sad. Maybe it was that she was growing up and I had lost my friend, or maybe it was just because I wanted everyone to believe, as I believe: that we were all one. Where we grew up and what problems the planet threw at us defined our culture, but ultimately I wanted to believe as always, that we were one. Our relationship changed after that and that is perhaps as it should be. Nothing in life, it would seem, is permanent.

Dr. Steichen, the chairman of surgery, developed squamous cell carcinoma of the throat and required operation. This affected his voice and his ability to speak, but not his spirit. I resented the other attendings for plotting against him behind his back. They suggested that he no longer was able to be chairman. Ultimately it was because they all wanted his job. The person most adamant about him not being physically able to perform his duties was the guy who had, in fact, done his surgery. That was my first lesson about jealousy amongst doctors. Unfortunately, that pattern of jealousy has shown through no matter where I've been. It's a part of medicine and life that I have come to hate. But it is a part of medicine and life that seems to always be there.

Lenox Hill Hospital, though, eventually put out a search for a new chairman. And lo and behold, those attendings that would undermine Dr. Steichen learned the lesson of their lives. Be careful what you wish for—you might get it. Dr. M. Michael Eisenberg arrived on the scene at Lenox Hill Hospital and his first order of business was to demonstrate to everyone that he was in fact in charge. He didn't need to be here, he chose it.

The most frightening moment for me was attending a conference, and a doctor came up to me and said, "I hear Dr. Eisenberg's with you guys now. Man, that guy's a bastard." And I thought, that must really be true, because this person doesn't know me. Dr. Eisenberg and I could be the best friends in the world. For him to say that without knowing me meant that he must really believe his assessment. Dr. Eisenberg, though, was not as bad as people tried to make him. He had a very hard time being friendly. He seemed uncomfortably around people. There was warmth lacking that I believe as surgeons we all had to have. But the real answer was we don't.

Dr. Eisenberg had taken over a job where there were residents in place that he had no part in choosing. He was determined to put his stamp on Lenox Hill Hospital. I tried as much as possible to establish a relationship with him, but it never seemed to take. You just could not trust that he was genuine, and any display of warmth on his part would quickly be followed by a coldness that would give you chills.

I chose to apply to plastic surgery programs without going through Dr. Eisenberg. All of the programs required a letter from your chairman. I chose Dr. Steichen write that letter rather than Eisenberg. He believed that to be a slap in the face and whatever chance we had of even being cordial went away with that, but I saw a letter that he had written for my co-chief resident, Dr. Morad Tavalalli. Morad was an Iranian national who had studied in London and the U.S. He had this awesome British accent. Morad worked as hard as anybody, and all Eisenberg could say about him was he had a great speaking voice.

And so I went about my application process without him. And lo, and behold, the University of Michigan accepted me. That was perhaps the biggest coup to this day in my medical career. The program at the University of Michigan was one of the best in the nation, and had a very proud history of medicine, including the Mayo brothers.

I had also interviewed at Wright State University in Dayton, Ohio. My intention was and always has been to one day return home to Middletown. Somehow I just never got around to it. I believe that my life is somehow less for that, but my hope is that I will get around to it before it's too late.

8

If you talk with physicians, they will tell you that "clearly you learn most of what you need to know about being a doctor after medical school." That is a fact. While med school gives you a platform, it's the interaction that you get from patients and other physicians that truly gives you your expertise. While there is a lot of information to be learned about the human body, the art of medicine really has to do with your investigative skills and your ability to put together a story. That transformation happened for me at the University of Michigan.

I owe most of my development as a physician to two people: David Smith, who was chairman of the division of Plastic surgery at U of M, and Riley Reese, who was his second in command. David Smith was from Indiana and his mannerisms and background demonstrated that. Having grown up on the Ohio-Indiana border, I got to know quite a number of people like David. He was smart, he was charming, and his background had afforded him an opportunity to know who he was. That's the advantage of growing up in small town Midwest. You get time to define yourself.

Riley was from the South, and you could hear it in every Southernism he used to explain medicine. "KISS," he would say all the time, "Keep It Simple, Stupid."

Michigan was a tremendous learning experience for me. My education there changed my life. David Smith and Riley Reese taught me how to think, instead of what to think. That is a gift for which I will forever be grateful.

Here's how it worked. Weekly, we had rounds where we discussed the patients and their treatment. As the chief resident on a particular service, it was your job to present the cases to the attending staff, other residents, and medical students, while Smith and Riley asked you questions about the care of a particular patient. It was not a friendly interchange.

Smith, regardless of how much information you had on a patient, knew how to probe, how to get to the question that you couldn't answer. You never got away without realizing there was always more to do. It was embarrassing. Remember, you have med students present who you're trying to impress as a good doctor and also trying to teach. To stand there in front of the group and have Smith dissect you was painful.

Riley Reese came to me after one of these sessions and laughing said, "Jan, why do you let David get you so flustered? You know more about the subject than he does." And a lot of times I believe I did. But David Smith truly knew how to think, not what to think, and that gave him an advantage. No matter what you had to say, there was always that next question that required an answer.

Interestingly, Smith really didn't care what you chose for a patient. He really didn't care how you went about caring for them. What Smith cared about most was that you knew why you were doing it? He required that you have at least five articles written in the plastic surgery literature that explained why you made the decision you made.

I soon learned to be even more thorough. Clearly one of the greatest accomplishments in our time has been the computer. It gives us the ability to be experts by searching for information around the globe in an instant. I would pull up obscure articles written in Russia, Romania, or France and have them translated to

English. I would then quote that study during one of Smith's sessions. The other residents would look at me in amazement. The answer, though, wasn't that I had done any more work. The answer was that I had learned the gift from Smith, and he in fact was a genius at it.

Speaking of the residents, the University of Michigan took three plastic surgery residents per year. That meant that there were a total of six of us in a two-year program. However, the year before me had only two. As a result, there were four of us my year. Dan, who started the program with us, had been the selection of the year before. He had chosen to hold off a year while he did research. I comment on that because we, the plastic surgery residents, worked much harder than most residents in heart surgery. I can't imagine how hard it was the previous year for the two guys ahead of us. The most grueling lesson was Smith's clinic. Smith saw about 100 people on his clinic day—that's right, 100. When you did his clinic, you had to see them all. Therefore, you saw 45 people in the morning prior to lunch and 55 afterwards.

Smith also taught me an important key about how you treat patients. Having to see 45 patients in about three hours meant that you didn't get to spend a lot of time with them, but you clearly had to make them feel that way. And so in my interactions with patients, I learned to do a few things: 1) I always sit down and never stand by the door; 2) regardless of what the patient has to say or I have to say, I always wait until the patient has completely finished and I allow for that awkward pause that occurs when people are done and we're just sitting there staring at each other; 3) I never look at my watch, and I always look the patient in the face; and 4) finally, you never touch the doorknob until you're ready to leave the room. That way, no matter how much time you spent with the patient, there was some completeness. That gave the patient the impression they had had enough time to say what they needed to say.

Managing people was Dr. Smith's forte, and he was a master. The greatest recollection I have of him was sitting in his office one day when his wife called. Dr. Smith had two sons, both in their early teens. That day Nancy called, not really to ask for any help, but to release some of the stress that accompanies raising two boys. You could hear her through the phone. Her speech was pressured, going on and on, not pausing between sentences, and certainly not pausing between paragraphs. On and on she went without taking a breath. After about three minutes of this, Smith calmly spoke into the phone and said, "Nancy, just tell me what you want me to do and I'll do it." Wham. There was complete silence at the other end of the phone. There's not much you can say to that. You could feel her calm down. You could feel her get control. I thought, "Wow, that's one to keep for the ages." If you do whatever someone else wishes, there's not much to add.

The biggest problem for any resident is getting everything done each day. There are people to see, things to read (to make sure that you were on top of patient care), and then there was the busy work, including the dictating of charts. It is the administrative work that would come back to haunt you if you didn't do it. At most hospitals, once a month medical records prints a delinquency list of those charts, and those residents responsible for them, that have not been completed. Normally our posture was to wait on this list and then, after having procrastinated as long as we could, be forced to go down and complete them.

Smith called me in the office one day and said, "JR, I want you to do me a favor. I want you to go down to the record room and find out who's responsible for the list of residents with delinquent charts. I want you to have him call you two days before he makes the list. And then, those two days before the list comes out, I want you to go down to the medical records office and dictate those charts." I never appeared on that list again. Smith's point was this: learn to use the system, don't let the system use you.

One of the best things about training at Michigan was the camaraderie between the residents. The four of us virtually did everything together. We arrived at the hospital around 5:30 and we spent the whole day together until we left at 7:30 or 8 pm that night. We got to know each other very well. It was comforting to know that it wasn't all just happening to you.

One of the moments of clarity for me occurred when Dan #1, who was really from the year before, talked about his family. Dan, Ed, and Dan #2 were married. I was not. Personally I think that was a prerequisite to get into the plastic surgery program at the University of Michigan and I somehow fell through the cracks. Dan commented on how hard we were working. It was brutal to go through the day, having people who had certainly more knowledge and expertise than you pound on you for what you did not know. In a sense he was correct. No one ever seemed to support you for what you did know. The cup was always half empty.

All Dan#2 talked about during the day was his two small girls, approximately three and four years old. What he said was this, "No matter how bad his day was, when he got home, there were two little girls who thought he was the greatest thing in the world. No matter how down he was, when he hit that door he was a happier person because of them." He offered that he felt bad for those of us, meaning me, who didn't have that experience: those of us who got home at the end of the day and merely had to confront that somehow that day you hadn't measured up. You didn't know all the answers. You didn't solve all the problems. And more than likely, you didn't get everything done that you wished you had gotten done.

That all changed when the next year of residents arrived. Noel was from New York, Steve was from Phoenix, and then there was Jeff, who you could characterize as nothing more (or less) than Smith cloned. It was clear that Jeff was going to be very successful.

Noel and I hit it off immediately. In a sense, he became my family. Most of our time away from the hospital was spent together. We talked about life, we'd complain about the workload, and we'd date nurses from the same nursing unit. That friendship has lasted to this day, and even now I consider him family, more than just a friend.

That second year began with one of the most frightening experiences I had had as a physician. A cute little six-year-old boy, blond hair, blue eyes, and helpless, was brought into Mott's Children's Hospital with meningitis. He arrived the day my second year began. I inherited him as my patient that day and spent the entire year with him. Meningitis can result in loss of integrity of the blood flow to different areas of the body, particularly the extremities. We watched helplessly as he began to lose toes, his foot, and then his lower legs. Every day I needed to change his bandages. It was difficult knowing that every day you were putting this kid through excruciating pain. I felt so bad for his mother and father having to watch this happen. Day in and day out, I'd round in the intensive care unit and work on this kid for about an hour.

He did get better and he did survive it, but the cost was the loss of his lower extremities. On the day that I finished my residency training at the University of Michigan, he was discharged home. His mother thanked me, made me a promise that she would stay in touch, and also that she would let me know from time to time how he was doing.

Michigan also provided one of my biggest joys. I had an uncle, Terrell Burton, who had coached football at Michigan with Bo Schembechler for 20 years. I hadn't been able to spend a lot of time with him because they lived so far away, but my Aunt Sue and my mother would speak all the time. Sue and Terrell were all about encouragement. Sue always had a smile and the best thing you can say about Terrell was that he was a coach. No matter when I got to see them, they were always loving and always giving—well that is, except one weekend a year. Once a year the University of Michigan played Ohio State University in football. Terrell, who knew I loved Ohio State football, would ride me for the whole week. I'd get calls at the hospital, where he'd say, "Watch out for this play. We're going to do this to you on Saturday."

Terrell invited me and the entire plastic surgery division to the training facility where the University of Michigan football team prepared for games each week. There were lecture halls, with motivational slogans on the walls, and indoor football fields. Let's just say that this group of doctors and nerds were literally in heaven. You could feel the history. You could feel the excitement that went along with University of Michigan football. It was simply great.

Also, at that time my training career was winding down. I was looking for what to do next. Do I go home to private practice? Do I continue on? Having been accepted to the University of Michigan training program meant that you would somehow go into academic medicine. No one said it, no one brought it up. It was just something that was expected.

I looked through the possibilities and found that Dr. Tim Miller at UCLA School of Medicine was establishing a fellowship in aesthetic surgery. As I mentioned earlier, there are four areas of plastic surgery: craniofacial, hand, reconstructive, and aesthetic surgery. Aesthetic surgery, while it gets all the press, really represents a small part of what plastic surgeons do. I knew immediately that this was the program for me. I discussed it with Riley who helped me do the necessary things to secure an application.

UCLA was slow in giving a decision, and both Riley and I struggled with the wait. Oddly enough, he could take it no more and he put in a call to UCLA to press the issue. I was awarded the fellowship. I was to be the first fellowship trained aesthetic surgeon to spend a year at a university-sponsored program. "Wow!"

9

As I headed west toward Los Angeles, I was filled with anticipation. There was tremendous excitement in what I was about to do. I had just completed my residency in plastic and reconstructive surgery at the University of Michigan, and I had completed it with a bang. Dr. Smith, during our graduation ceremonies, had offered that during the first year when he watched me do my work, he thought I was the best black resident he'd ever had. However, at the graduation dinner, he offered that Jan was in fact not the best black resident he had ever had; he was in fact the best resident he'd ever had.

Dr. Warren Garner, who was the youngest member of the staff, pulled me aside to reassure me that that was in no way a racial slur. Personally, I hadn't taken it as that. I had taken it as nothing but positive. But that was Dr. Warren Garner. When you first met Warren, you thought he was prissy and particular. It turned out after you'd spent enough time with him that what lie below was a meticulous plastic surgeon who had the kindest heart of any of us, myself included.

Warren always made sure, with an off-the-cuff statement here or there, that you could be doing better; that there were certain things that were unacceptable and you needed to pay attention to detail. And no matter where he was when he ran into you, and no matter what was going on, he made sure that he gave you that dig, just to remind you. But nonetheless, he was someone who you could always trust, you knew where he was coming from, and ultimately he had your best interest at hand.

And so my drive west was indeed exciting. I looked forward to seeing Steve Crisman, a friend from New York and visiting with his wife, Marielle Hemingway, and their daughters. They offered the family and the stability that I was to need when I got to L.A. I just really appreciated them being there.

After saying my hellos and spending a couple of days with them, I headed up the coast to Malibu to find a place to live. I settled on a condominium that sat on a hill on the east side of Pacific Coast Highway. The complex looked down on the famed Colony where all the movie stars lived, and then out onto the ocean. This apartment was perfectly located. Just below was the shopping center at the Colony with a grocery store, custom shops, postal service, and a service station. The government buildings for Malibu City services were also just below, about half a mile south. The complex was perfect and it offered everything I needed, at least so I thought.

The drive to UCLA took approximately 25 minutes each morning, and it was this drive that taught me something very interesting. Living at the extreme western part of the city is probably not a good idea. During the first two months or so, I seemed to always keep a headache. I couldn't figure out why. Then one day it dawned on me. When I went to work in the morning, the sun was in my face, and as I returned home that evening, the sun was once again directly in my face. I resolved then to live on the east side of the city and head west or when I'm finished with this program, return to the East Coast.

Regardless, there would be plenty of time to think about those things. I was now the Aesthetic Fellow in Plastic and Reconstructive Surgery at the UCLA Medical Center.

Orientation was confusing. I was the pioneer and the one setting the tone for the Fellowship. There were a lot of the details that were open and had to be defined by me. Dr. Miller's office was in the newer outpatient surgery center at 200 UCLA Medical Plaza. Across the street was the massive UCLA Medical Center, including the Neuropsychological Hospital, the UCLA Hospital, the Children's Hospital, and various clinics. That was a maze that I wanted to avoid. And so, I tried as much as possible to confine the workings of the Fellowship to 200 UCLA Medical Plaza.

I began by first proceeding to the chairman's office to get the prospectus for the year. That included the Division of Plastic Surgery anatomy sessions, the Saturday morning workshops, and the UCLA Division of Plastic and Reconstructive Surgery grand rounds schedule. Once these were recorded, it was then time to arrange my schedule. I wanted to allow myself as much time as possible to spend with the physicians who would take part in the program, and the residents who I would help with surgeries and clinics.

Tim and I sat down first and to the surprise, I think, of many in the department, we immediately hit it off. Tim was considered withdrawn and intellectual. I found him to be that, but I also found him to be warm and caring. I knew he had wanted this Fellowship to succeed, and it was to that end that I dedicated myself.

The staff at UCLA was actually quite impressive. Dr. William Shaw, who was the chairman, had come from NYU and was quite famous for microsurgical techniques. Even more impressive was the casual clinical staff. They were the plastic and reconstructive surgeons in private practice in Beverly Hills and Santa Monica. This included Steve Hoefflin who had been Michael Jackson's surgeon, Jack Sheen who had written the book on nose surgery, Henry Kawamoto who pretty much had defined craniofacial surgery in America, and John Williams who in the early '60s had defined cosmetic plastic surgery.

I loved John Williams. In spite of all his expertise, and literally all of his fame as a cosmetic surgeon, at seventy years of age he was more than willing to learn and try anything new. And that's exactly the reason I went into plastic and reconstructive surgery. As a medical student, hearing plastic surgeons explain that this procedure was one they had never been done before was fascinating. They were, in fact, going to evaluate the anatomy and devise an operation that specifically solved the needs of that patient. I loved it. It wasn't about learning operations and trying to mold the patient to fit. It was about understanding the patient's problems and devising an operation that worked for them. It was perfect for me; it was perfect for how I thought.

As the Fellowship started, I began as an outcast. Everyone was uncertain of exactly what to expect. Gradually the residents and attendings began to warm up. The first three months were actually tremendous fun. I was running conferences, I was helping the residents with their clinic, and I was doing surgery on my own patients with me making all the decisions, and yet there was comfort in knowing that in the next room was someone there if I needed help.

This cruised along for another month, and then things began to change. More and more of the clinical staff began to question the necessity of a fellowship in cosmetic surgery. They weren't really sure why we needed one. I was confused by that posture. There was a fellowship in microsurgery. There was a fellowship in craniofacial surgery. There were even fellowships in hand surgery.

Obviously I agreed with Dr. Miller that there should also be a fellowship in cosmetic surgery. This is why I was there. We, as plastic surgeons, were expected to do the best cosmetic surgery. It only seemed natural that we should be the best trained in it. Besides, there was certainly a lot of animosity over the fact that gynecologists had started doing liposuction, ophthalmologists had started doing more eyelid surgery, and ENT people actually began to call themselves facial plastic surgeons.

Many plastic surgeons felt that their area was being infringed upon and they resented it. My concern, however, was that their resentment was misdirected. Their frustration was not directed at those people whom they thought were infringing on their rights.

Their anger did not motivate them to be better at it. They began to do the absolute incorrect thing. They began to fight amongst themselves.

As is the case with most institutions, they crumble from within, not from without. Dr. Miller's Aesthetic Fellowship became the first thing for the clinical faculty to attack. They were more concerned that if they helped train too many people with more expertise at cosmetic surgery than they had, then eventually they, in some manner, would be below the standard of care. This was indeed a very short-sighted conclusion.

The clinical staff began to fabricate reasons for needing to dissolve the fellowship: It was too time-consuming. It required that the resident train too long. They began to question whether the program itself was economically feasible. Nonetheless, I was able to demonstrate that the Aesthetic Fellowship had in fact earned more money than it had cost to pay me. It actually began to chip away at the enthusiasm with which I began the job. I was devastated that the faculty was actually killing a program because it raised the standard of care.

By the time May had rolled around, they had actually succeeded in undermining the program. Even though there was a resident who had signed up to follow, you could tell that the program did not have much of a future. I resented that. My immediate reaction was to isolate myself from this group. I would prove to them that I was a better surgeon. I was determined to treat my patients better than any of them treated theirs.

I decided that once I started my practice, I would do my work and go home. I would limit my interaction with colleagues to the absolute minimum. I would as much as possible avoid the politics and petty jealousies. I knew to isolate myself from this group, my colleagues, was career wise not the smartest thing to do, but once again, people had demonstrated to me that they were best avoided. I refused to live the rest of my life looking over my shoulder watching to see which plastic surgeon would be the one to stick a knife in my back.

10

THE DECISION TO PARTICIPATE IN A TV SHOW WAS MORE desperation than inspiration. When I finished at UCLA, the hard question once again was whether to pursue a career in academic medicine or to go into private practice. In a sense, fate answered that for me. Medicine was experiencing, from an economic standpoint, a drastic slowdown. As a result, those people who had entered into academic positions, who normally would have matriculated into private practice, were no longer doing so. They were holding onto those jobs because they offered security.

I put a call into my former chairman, Dave Smith, to discuss my options. His first inclination was that I should look for an academic job. My other alternative of course was to pursue a career in private practice. I was offered a position as an associate of John Williams.

John Williams was the premier plastic surgeon of his time. In a sense his career had defined cosmetic plastic surgery, particularly in southern California. I enjoyed the moments I spent talking with him. He'd often reminisce about the good old days when celebrities or movie stars would come into his office, lay down \$20,000 or \$30,000, and ask him to fix them. In today's world, from his perspective, that had changed drastically. The patients were now coming in telling him what they wanted him to do, describing how he should do it, demanding that they pay him less, and yet, at the same time, wanting him to take the responsibility for the outcome. Somehow this seemed backwards, just plain wrong.

Many times, in our very private conversations, he'd suggest that for the long term I consider doing other things. He thought that the future of plastic surgery was bleak. He just thought that people were getting more selfish and mean and that the 'good old days' of plastic surgery were gone. I chalked it up to progress, but now I believe John was right. It was not sentiment on his part, it was observation.

John Williams believed my future my lie in media. In particular, he appreciated the fact that I was able to explain very complicated medical issues in layman's terms. Our office, Aesthetica, was at 5757 Wilshire Boulevard in the same building that housed the offices of the Screen Actors Guild. Across the street were the offices for E, Entertainment Television.

Aesthetica, as an office, was beautiful. It was modern, tastefully done with soft pink colors, and a tremendous office staff that screamed success. John's brother Jim had worked with him at one time; in fact, they were twins. Jim's practice, however, never really took off to the extent of John's practice, but it was obvious as to why. No client was going to walk in off the street for plastic surgery and choose you, meaning any other doctor, knowing that John Williams was next door.

Garth Fischer, who had finished at UC Irvine a couple of years earlier, had also taken a position as an associate with John. Garth proved helpful because of his insight into getting a practice started. He seemed comfortable at Aesthetica, and so I settled in and began the task of creating a private practice.

Things went wonderfully at first, as all the people who were waiting for you to complete training began having procedures done. But realistically, after you'd completed surgery on all your mother's friends, it was now time to get going. The real game was now on.

In one conversation with John, we talked about how, in the past as a physician, you could go into a bank and get the funds needed to start a practice. In today's world, that was clearly not going to happen. Many plastic surgeons, particularly the older ones, were retiring because they were unable to make ends meet. In the long run, it just wasn't worth it for them to be spending money out of pocket to survive if they weren't producing the volume to replace that money. I solved it by covering emergency rooms throughout the South Bay. I had received a call from Dr. Pearlman Hicks, down in Long Beach, whose wife unfortunately had developed breast cancer. After her death, he was looking for a way to spend more time with his children. I consented to cover his call schedule so that he would have more time for his boys.

And so, in addition to Aesthetica, I became a staff member at approximately 12 hospitals in the South Bay. At first it was almost comical. I would be at the emergency room at Long Beach Memorial at 3 a.m. Friday/Saturday morning, and at the same time get a call to sew up the face of an accident victim at Downey Hospital approximately 20 miles away. The weekends were spent driving from one hospital to the next sewing up lacerations, repairing hand fractures, and attending to accident victims.

At first, as I said, it was comical because it was fun. After a few months, it became tedious, especially since you started to realize that the insurance companies were not only paying you 10-20¢ on the dollar, but many times not paying at all. I attempted to solve this problem by using an independent billing service, International Medical Financials. I met its owner and heard his pitch. They were representing hundreds of doctors. I believed that the billing would be standardized and as such would be paid in a timely fashion. Eight months went by before small checks started to trickle in.

Also by that time I was seeing patients in follow-up on Tuesday afternoons from 2 to 5 in the office of Dr. Hicks. It seemed unfair to ask some of these people who were general laborers to drive all the way to Beverly Hills. Since Dr. Hicks' office was centrally located, I thought it easier that I pick a day and see them down there. It worked fine at first and then became an economic issue. Dr. Hicks began billing me for a third of his office's overhead but I didn't have an office there. For the three hours once a week that I went there, I worked out of a nurse's station and basically saw only follow-ups; and even with that, I was paying his office 50% of the revenue.

That apparently wasn't enough for him, and the bills for a third of his overhead kept coming. I met with Dr. Hicks and explained to him that I did not have an office here. I pointed out that I was working at his request so that he could spend time with his children. Furthermore, we had never talked about me joining his practice or paying him for a third of his overhead. Also, 100% of this money was insurance money, and he was already in fact getting half.

This continued for a few months. It became apparent that as medicine economically continued to shrink, things here weren't going to get better. I severed my relationship with Dr. Hicks, opting to set up my own office in Beverly Hills. Dr. Williams also was considering retirement and the time seemed right to go out on my own.

Precisely one month after I had moved to Beverly Hills, I received a summons from Dr. Hicks' attorney suing me for a third of his overhead over the 12 months that I had covered for him. Dr. Hicks, by the way, was my uncle: no act of kindness goes unpunished. And oh … there was that knife I was talking about.

The move to Beverly Hills was exciting. In spite of all that was going on around me bad, I kept looking forward toward the future. Yes, medicine was changing, things were getting harder, but I continued to believe that they would get better as long as I persevered. Besides, according to the calculations of International Medical Financials, I had accumulated accounts receivables of approximately $387,000 over that year and a half. Unfortunately, also by their calculations in that period, I had received only about $80,000 in payment of which $40,000 went to Dr. Hicks. It was very obvious that something different had to happen.

It started with a call from a woman who was a segment producer for a TV show. As part of my advertising, I was lecturing to different groups in the community. She had heard me give a talk on plastic surgery, and was working on a variety show where they needed a plastic surgeon to talk about wrinkles. Her name was Sharon Nash, and I liked her immediately. Our call went something like this: "Dr. Jan, this is Sharon Nash. I'm doing a TV show and we need a plastic surgeon to talk about wrinkles. I was wondering if you would do that." I thought for a second and then quickly told her no. There was silence at the other end. For her I imagine this was unbelievable. Who wouldn't want to be on TV? We exchanged niceties. I hung up and went back to my day.

The next day I got a call from her and this time she made her pitch. "Look," she said, "I'm the only black girl working on this show. We've got a big problem finding a plastic surgeon to talk about wrinkles. If you do it, it will help me." And so I accepted.

I went down to the studios at Universal two days later. It was a variety show put on by Jake Steinfeld of Body by Jake fame. I didn't get to meet Jake until we were on stage, but it was clear that I was not what he was expecting. "Ladies and gentlemen," he said, "Let me introduce a Beverly Hills plastic surgeon, Dr. Jan Adams." Well, I walked out on the stage and Jake stumbled back. He wasn't expecting a 6'3" tall black guy with a shaved head. Jake and I exchanged hellos. I talked about wrinkling from an anatomical standpoint and specific treatments.

After the show, the producer approached me and said, "You're funny."

I apologized for anything that I'd done that was wrong.

"Oh, no," she said, "You didn't do anything wrong. I sit behind the audiences when we are taping and the women in the audience loved you. You might consider doing this." I thought momentarily and declined. But TV people can be persistent, and after about a week I received a call from this executive producer.

"Dr. Jan," she said, "I want you to do a demo tape."

"OK," I said, "What's a demo tape?"

"A demo tape is where you get in front of a camera and you talk about yourself for about five minutes."

"Five minutes," I said. "I could talk about myself forever."

She chuckled and offered that I didn't need to do it forever. Five minutes would be more than enough. We arranged the taping and I did the demo tape.

According to the cameraman, I apparently was a natural. It seems that it's generally very difficult for people to stand in front of a camera and talk about themselves without stuttering or falling over the words. The only people who had done as well as he had seen me do it were radio people. They have been trained to avoid dead air. You can't see someone on the radio, and so they have to be talking all the time. At any rate, that demo tape made it to USA Studios and I found myself in a meeting with one of the producers there who signed me to a development contract.

Simultaneously, a close friend of mine, Thom Beeres, of Original Productions fame, was interested in producing a show for Discovery Networks. He and I met at the Newsroom Café on Robertson in Beverly Hills and literally wrote the treatment for a plastic surgery show on napkins. "Plastic Surgery: Before and After," we would call it. We would tell stories about people using preoperative and postoperative photos of them as the payoff. It was a great idea on Tom's part. Plastic surgery lent itself exactly to a visual presentation. I'd even shared with him that "when people come to the office, the one thing they all want to do is look at before and after pictures." Even those people who were impatient, and in a hurry to get in and out, seemed to find the time to browse when it came to those booklets of photos.

Also, NBC Studios was looking for talent to star in a show which would be the male version of "The View."

We were unable at USA Studios to come up with a project, and when I was free of that commitment I interviewed for the job on a show was to be known as "The Other Half." It starred Dick Clark, Danny Bonaduce, myself, and Mario Lopez. I learned a lot about television from Dick Clark. The most important thing to understand was that when you're talking to that camera, you're really only talking to one person. So relax and have a conversation with them. That was key. It gave me a comfort; that helped me a lot in that career.

I lasted only one season. The concept didn't seem to fly. The executive producer came to me and said, "Jan, I need you to do me a favor."

I thought, "Of course."

"Well," she said, "I need you not to know the answer. Some of the affiliates think you talk down to the other guys and I just need you to not know the answers sometimes."

"How could I not know the answer? I asked. You've got Bonaduce at the other end of the podium screaming, 'you're Dr. Jan, a Harvard-educated plastic surgeon.' How can I look stupid under those circumstances? Besides, I'm not talking down to them. We're all playing roles here. I'm supposedly the sophisticated professional."

In actuality, it turned out that the affiliates—those who owned the stations—were uncomfortable with the black guy being the reasonable one. Psychologically, that was devastating for me. I thought we had clearly evolved past that, but I guess we hadn't.

Going full circle, I was now available to do "Plastic Surgery: Before and After" on Discovery Health Channel. That also brings us full circle to the problem that I had not anticipated. The problem: other plastic surgeons.

If you called me and said, "I have this or that symptom, what should I do?" it would be very easy for me to address. However, I'm not sure how you deal with other people's jealousy. If you treat them well, they say you're condescending. If you avoid them, they say you're stuck up. "Plastic Surgery: Before and After" really made me a target. Every plastic surgeon who thought it should be him, or her, rather than me on TV explaining plastic surgery procedures, essentially saw me as the target. There were the occasional interactions where people were happy that someone had put plastic surgery in such an honorable and academic light, but those people were few. The majority of plastic surgeons across America would call the offices and offer to debate Jan on issues concerning plastic surgery. Unfortunately for me, it was creating enemies I didn't even know I had.

Incidentally, it's important to note that all of this took place before the issues of DUI's, divorce, malpractice suits or the Medical Board of California. In fact, in terms of malpractice suits and the Medical Board of California I would argue that TV was in fact the cause.

I mention this because it's very important to put a time frame on what Harvey Levin was saying on Larry King Live. In his interview Harvey Levin opined, "But, Larry, What's interesting about this is that he was on "The Oprah Winfrey Show" almost as the go to plastic surgeon. He was on the Discovery Channel. He was on NBC on a show they had there. And no one-none of this, none of this surfaced. And, clearly, you know, had they known, this would have raised a red flag in terms of putting him on the show because it's almost like a Good Housekeeping stamp of approval."

I'm concerned for Harvey because once again he demonstrates his laziness, or his stupidity. None of this showed up at that time because none of it had happened at that time. My casting for these shows took place in 2000, 2001, and 2002. The acquittal of the DUI, and the conviction for a BAL greater than. 08 took place in 2006. By the way, "Plastic Surgery: Before and After" had been cancelled already. Its five years were up. Oprah could not have considered it because it hadn't happened. Give Oprah a break.

And certainly for completion's sake take a look at all these so-called malpractice suits. You'll see they coincide with my decision to try and help those people who otherwise would not be able to afford plastic surgery. You see, the guy on TV, the go-to guy, makes an easy target.

I was proud of "Plastic Surgery: Before and After", at least until the tragic death of Donda West. It was at that time that the PR people at Discovery Networks called (for the first time in six years) and asked that I don't mention them should I go on Larry King

Live. They were distancing themselves from me before they had even heard my side of the story. Donald Thoms, a vice president in charge of production at Discovery Health and someone I love, disappeared.

And yet, one of our major sponsors was the American Society of Plastic and Reconstructive Surgery. They paid to advertise the services of their members to the general public on our show. Not once, in five years of programming, had anyone from their organization challenged any of the information I shared. They all wanted to be on the show, but they could not find fault with us (or me) and surely most of their members tried.

In terms of private practice, John Williams' predictions had been correct. People were more demanding, less inclined to be happy with results, and just meaner. I grew increasingly unhappy.

I searched for other alternatives including reducing the amount of time that I spent in the office doing plastic surgery. Every day got to be too much. At a certain level, I was beginning not to like the patients. That was more devastating than any other factor. I needed these people. I wanted to help them. It was important for me to help them in order to feel good about myself.

A friend of mine offered an alternative. Raad Jeroudi is an anesthesiologist with a vision. His plan was to provide surgery at an affordable price. He wanted to offer great surgery, no frills. My job would only be to do surgery. I would come in, evaluate a patient, discuss procedures with them, schedule them for surgery, do the surgery, and then do the follow-up. His office would do all the administrative work like schedule appointments, do the paperwork, collect the money, and act as a liaison between the doctor and the patient.

This worked wonderfully, but soon we became victims of our own success. There were more patients than time could accommodate. The patients, even though they were getting cut rates to do premium surgery, were becoming more impatient and more demanding. There were constant threats of malpractice suits because patients had to wait an hour or two to be seen. Things like infections became malpractice rather than an unfortunate mishap. Hypertrophic scarring, which is known in women of color, became something the doctor did rather than a known complication of healing in people of color.

It did, however, inspire us to take a critical look at what we were doing. I reviewed 530 cases that we had done from July 2006 to June 2007. In that time period, there had been four infections. The national average for infections is 3%, which meant that statistically we should have at least 16. We had experienced only four, which was a fourth of that. Yet all four of these people were threatening malpractice suits. For me, that was more than enough. If I was going to have to deal with people who were angry, and wanted to see themselves as victims, then I would return to my old fee scale. I was not going out of my way to perform these procedures on people who otherwise might not be able to afford them, and then be wrongfully threatened each day. (Hence, Harvey Levin's "malpractice suit after malpractice suit" comments.) With that, I returned to Brentwood and solo practice.

With all that being said, I don't need to make excuses or apologize for who I am. No amount of unwarranted or malicious attacks on the part of the media is going to diminish what I stand for. I'm not going to apologize for a less than perfect life. I know that I am granted forgiveness by God to keep on trying to live a grander version, period.

With that having been said, let's get back to the coroner's report and see if we can put together Dr. West's post-operative course. We need to understand what happened in order to affect closure. I think Donda West deserves that (despite the fact that her nephew and his entertainment lawyers want to move on).

11

"DR. WEST'S DEATH WAS NOT THE RESULT OF ANESTHESIA OR surgery mishaps", that's Ed Winter, assistant-chief Investigator for the LA County Coroner's office speaking, not me. Earlier I attributed that statement to the Los Angeles County coroner. However, it should be understood that that is not his conclusion alone. The lead investigator, Dr. Louis Pena, consulted with other pathologists including those at UCLA and the University of Southern California. I might also add that at my request, the West family obtained their own pathologist to monitor this process. He was in agreement with the coroner's findings also. And so, the question at hand still remains, what really happened to Donda West?

Again, the answer rests somewhere in the coroner's report and it's important to analyze that.

According to her nephew, the nurse taking care of her when she was out of my direct care, the next morning she felt 100% better, so much so, that he felt comfortable in leaving her in the care of her assistant, Nubia, and her friend, Diana. (Although I still think it's important never to lose sight of the fact that he told the Coroner's investigator a lie saying "they were caregivers, referred by Dr. Adams".) Clearly the final cause of death is cardiopulmonary arrest meaning that her heart and lungs stopped working.

Despite the fact that the literature surrounding this case is riddled with the conclusion of a heart attack, neither the macroscopic nor the microscopic evaluations of her heart muscle, according to Dr. Pena demonstrate infarcts (i.e. injury to the muscle itself). The question is why her heart stopped? She had survived the surgery (for which Dr. Aboolian wanted her to have clearance). What happened in the time in which she was "100% better" according to her nephew and the calamity that was her 911 call?

Well, the first thing that happened was that her caregiver, an experienced nurse with an advanced degree, abandoned her to the care of her personal assistant and a friend neither of whom had any medical training. He did so without notifying her physician, or obtaining another qualified caregiver (nurse) to cover him.

According to Diana in an interview with *Sister2Sister* magazine (May, 2008) "Scoggins had been giving her pain medicine all night, but it wasn't working" (according to Donda). So at the very least, at the time this "experienced nurse with an advanced degree" made the decision to abandon his aunt, he knew she had a lot of the narcotic, Vicodin, in her system.

The coroner's report does note that there was vomitus in her lungs. This gives us a place in which to start. Vomitus in her lungs means that some degree of aspiration took place. Aspiration refers to sucking abdominal contents out of the stomach, up the esophagus, and then back down into the trachea and bronchi, and finally into the lung itself. In order for this to happen, there has to be some degree of paralysis of her gag reflex, which is the cough we all experience when a finger is placed too far to the back of our throat.

More specifically then, the question becomes, what came first—her heart stopping or the aspiration? If a "heart attack" appeared first, one would think she would have experienced some chest pain and would have either sat up' or cried out in pain. But the history, at least as given to the coroner, suggests that she didn't. No one heard her cry out, and when they found her, she was cold, clammy, and unresponsive.

If she was awake and aspirated first, then clearly there would have been an episode of coughing as she tried to clear her throat. But again, she didn't, because no one heard her. (Perhaps they would have, if her nephew, "an experienced nurse with an advanced degree" had obtained the monitors he said had when he arrived late to the surgery center to take her home. Surely, something as simple as a pulse oximeter, would have alerted even people in another room that she had stopped breathing.)

In order for her to aspirate abdominal contents into her lungs without attempting to sit up, she had to be asleep or passed out due to the Vicodin, her pain medication. The side effects of narcotics like Vicodin include decreased respirations, nausea, and loss of her gag reflex. (It is important to remember that all medications—in spite of being advertised on TV, prescribed freely, and taken with abandon—are very powerful drugs whose side effects can be disastrous. In fact, the unfortunate death of actor Heath Ledger is proof of that. It is painfully obvious that anesthesia and/or surgery are not a prerequisite for this to happen.)

The fact that the coroner reports vomitus in her lungs suggests that ASPIRATION was the inciting event.

From a medical standpoint, the rest is fairly easy to explain. Following aspiration of vomitus into the lungs, a ventilation perfusion inequality resulted and the blood began to decrease in oxygen tension. That means that having foreign material in your lungs causes the lungs to shift blood flow away from that area, thereby mixing it with oxygenated blood and lowering the total amount of oxygen in the blood that is therefore carried to the heart. As this process continued, the oxygen content of the blood continued to decrease.

Finally, as a result of the combination of respiratory arrest and the ventilation perfusion inequality, her heart stopped because it was not getting enough oxygen. (Again, you don't need underlying heart disease or surgery for this process to run its course.)

Interestingly, as reported by the coroner and confirmed by the patient and her nephew, a cardiac workup at Cedars-Sinai Medical Center, one of the premier cardiac hospitals in America, confirmed no heart disease. That, however, does not mean that she could not have had underlying changes in her heart that were consistent with her age. As a result, I believe the coroner's assessment is indeed accurate. What we have witnessed is a cardiac arrest resulting from a myriad of factors, the greatest of which would appear to be the aspiration of vomitus with subsequent decrease in oxygenation.

Despite the coroner's report that her post-mortem values for Vicodin were not elevated, I would caution that the samples were obtained at least two days after her death (we now know that individual cells continue to perform their functions even after the whole organism may be pronounced dead). She had vomited and certainly this would have decreased the amount of drug available for absorption. However, different people react differently to the same amount of drug (tolerance).

What I do know is that approximately one week after her death I received a frantic call from one of the women present in the home at the time of Dr. West's death.

Diana Pinckney had placed Dr. West's medications in her purse to show to the doctors at Centinela Marina Hospital. No one had asked for them and so she forgot they were there. She discovered them a week later while changing purses.

Of significance was at this time there were eight capsules of the antibiotic Keflex and 10 Vicodin tablets. She had been dispensed 10 Keflex and 30 Vicodin by the pharmacist. This means that in the period since she arrived home the night before at around 8 pm and 6 pm the next day, approximately 22 hours, Dr. West received 20 Vicodin tablets, almost three times the daily recommended dosage (So perhaps Ms Pinckney was correct in repeating from Donda that "Scoggins had been feeding me Vicodin all night".)

This was confirmed in a conversation with the coroner's office by telephone. A nurse in the coroner's office confirmed that this report was consistent with the history presented by other parties she had interviewed.

The question therefore remains: Where was her "experienced nurse with an advanced degree"?

12

WHEN ASKED FOR COMMENTS BY A NUMBER OF REPORTERS including those at *People* and *Sister2Sister* magazines, Stephan Scoggins replied that the family had no comment. They have, in fact, moved on. Yet if that were the case, then articles like the one that appeared in the Los Angeles times Sunday, May 25, 2008 would cease to appear. In that article, a niece comments that Ms. West surgery was performed without a physical exam. The author, Rong-Wong Lin II, suggests, correctly, the ludicrousness of the statement by pointing out that both the surgeon and the anesthesiologist examined Donda West. The niece goes on to point out that what happened to Donda didn't have to happen. She's right, but for the wrong reason. Just the silliness of her statement demonstrates that she doesn't have a clue about what happened to Donda, and who could move on under those circumstances.

The Coroner, along with experts from UCLA, USC, and the West family's own pathologist have ruled that "neither anesthesia nor surgery mishaps" caused Donda's death. Donda survived the surgery. Donda was home.

What Mr. Scoggins really means when he says "the family has moved on" is that he doesn't want to get into a discussion about what really happened. Ultimately that would mean looking at his own behavior, and neither he nor the lawyers involved want that. They also don't want the rest of the family (or the media) to take a critical look at the events leading up to Donda West's death.

Ask Mr. Scoggins why his aunt chose not to go to an aftercare facility? Ask Mr. Scoggins, an experienced nurse with an advanced degree, if he did not convince her to have surgery by assuring her that he would be there throughout the process (when in fact, her fear had caused her to cancel with other doctors many times before)? Ask Mr. Scoggins if he insisted she sign an "advanced directive" giving power to him? Ask Mr. Scoggins, an experienced nurse with an advanced degree, why he was late picking his aunt up? Ask Mr. Scoggins where the bed, the wheel chair, and the monitors he ordered for her aftercare were when they arrived home after surgery? Ask Mr. Scoggins, an experienced nurse with an advanced degree, why the monitors didn't even arrive the next morning as he assured everyone they would? Ask Mr. Scoggins, an experienced nurse with an advanced degree, why he abandoned his aunt the next morning? Ask Mr. Scoggins, an experienced nurse with an advanced degree, why he would abandon a patient whom he had been "feeding Vicodin all night and it wasn't working" to the care of her personal assistant and a friend, neither of whom had any medical training whatsoever? Ask Mr. Scoggins why he didn't check back all day? Ask Mr. Scoggins, an experienced nurse with an advanced degree, why he ignored their calls all day Saturday? Ask Mr. Scoggins, an experienced nurse with an advanced degree, how, on his watch, Donda West's medications demonstrated that she had received 20 Vicodin tabs in less than 24 hours, three times the daily recommended dose?

Ask Mr. Scoggins, an experienced nurse with an advanced degree, and the "so-called" lawyers for the estate, Mr. Brad Rose and Ed Mcpherson, why they don't release the doctor from the doctor-patient privilege and discuss the case in an open, and fair forum? (By the way, Kanye West and Shawn Gee were named co-executers of her will on May 29, 2008. At the time of her death, November 10, 2007, Donda West did not have a will. Mr. Rose and Mr. McPherson had been misrepresenting themselves all along.) Ask Mr. Scoggins why he took over discussing Donda's case with the authorities the night of her death, excluding Diana and Nubia, when they were the ones who had been there all day and he had not? Ask that niece Mr. Rong- Wong Lin II why the family doesn't insist on that discussion?

I don't know the answers to all those questions, but I do know that Mr. Scoggins and the so-called lawyers for the estate of Donda West were poised to crucify me and the Brentwood Surgery Center had the coroner ruled otherwise. I do know that they had (improperly) alerted the Medical Board of California, the California Department of Health Services, and the City Attorney's Office. I do know their intention was to implement us in Donda's death and thereby divert any attention from Mr. Scoggins. I do know that their plans were ruined when the coroner's report, along with independent examiners and the family's own pathologist, ruled that I had made no mishaps that led to her death.

I do know the press wanted to blame somebody—the surgeon being the most obvious—but everyone, it seemed, ignored the facts of the case. Donda West died at home, not the Brentwood Surgery Center. Donda West, it would seem, died as a result of gross negligence on the part of her nephew, an experienced nurse with an advanced degree. No sensible human being could arrive at any other conclusion.

Contrary to what the press would have us believe, Donda West was scheduled for a post-operative care facility with experienced nurses like him. I can guarantee you that none of them would have left her alone for 12 hours with her personal assistant and a friend; no nurse would have left her alone without certainly calling her doctor or passing her care along to another nurse. No nurse I know would have abandoned their patient and relative in order to attend a baby shower less than 12 hours after her surgery. No nurse I know would have abandoned his or her patient and then ignored calls all day from the people with whom he left her, ultimately turning off his phone so as not to be bothered. No nurse I know would have left his aunt alone all day less than 24 hours after surgery and arrived at the hospital after her death, already pointing fingers at the other women in the house.

Mr. Scoggins didn't point fingers at me at the time—no, he didn't even express regret. The first words out of Stephan's mouth to me were, "Can you believe that there were three women in the house and none of them were with her?" Yes, Mr. Scoggins, the experienced nurse with the advanced degree, had already begun making sure no one evaluated his behavior in this matter. Even with me on the night of Donda's death he was blaming Nubia, Diana, and Glenda, her best friend.

I cautioned him, "Frankly, we don't know what happened here yet. We, you and I, are the only medical professionals here. Let's don't do things that are going to further hurt this family. Let's you and I be supportive."

I then walked with him to the nurse's station to sign the death certificate. The real answer, however, is that he was the medical professional contracted to care for her for the entire weekend and he wasn't with her either.

But what was to happen in the next few days is even more telling. Stephan Scoggins, a nurse, who according to his own website is a former police officer from the State of Oklahoma, lied to the LA County Coroner. Then, along with the help of Donda West's estate's (which did not exist) attorneys, Mr. Brad Rose of Pryor Cashman in New York City and Edwin McPherson of Los Angeles began to orchestrate a series of events to cover up Stephan's involvement.

Never forget that these people are entertainment lawyers first, who are adept at publicity and getting a story out the way they want it told. Mr. Rose was the first to get involved. I received a letter from him Tuesday morning that was accusatory and mean.

-2007 03:21pm From-PRYOR CASHMAN LLP +12123260806 T-517 P.002/003 F-600

PRYOR CASHMAN LLP New York | Los Angeles

410 Park Avenue, New York, NY 10022 Tel: 212-421-4100 Fax: 212-326-0806 www.pryorcashman.com

Brad D. Rose
Partner

Direct Tel: 212-326-0875
Direct Fax: 212-798-6369
brose@pryorcashman.com

November 13, 2007

VIA FEDERAL EXPRESS & FACSIMILE

Jan R. Adams, M.D.
450 North Bedford Drive
Beverly Hills, CA 90212

Re: Dr. Donda West

Dear Dr. Adams:

This office, together with McPherson & Associates, are litigation counsel to the Estate of Dr. Donda West and the surviving personal representatives of Dr. West. It has come to our attention that you or your office have been disseminating private medical information about Dr. West as well as medical advice that was allegedly imparted within the context of the physician/patient relationship that existed between you and Dr. West.

As you well know, under California and Federal law, the fact of any consultations or meetings that Dr. West may have had with you, together with the substance of those consultations/meetings, clearly constitute private, confidential, and privileged communications. Under relevant California and Federal authority, the physician/patient privilege survives the untimely passing of Dr. West, and can and will continue to be asserted by Dr. West's personal representatives, the "holders" of that privilege under California Evidence Code Section 993 (c), whom we also represent.

Specifically, TMZ.com has reported that you told them the following:

"Plastic surgeon Dr. Jan Adams has told TMZ that he was the doctor who performed cosmetic surgery on Kanye West's mother Donda before she died. "Dr. Adams told TMZ her death, which followed a tummy tuck and breast reduction, was unforeseen and could have been caused by a heart attack, pulmonary embolism, or massive vomiting. "Dr. Adams tells TMZ West consulted with him over a period of four months. He says she changed her mind numerous times, sometimes greenlighting the surgery and sometimes halting it."

Figure 24

-2007 03:21pm From-PRYOR CASHMAN LLP +12123260806 T-517 P.003/003 F-600

PR'OR CASHMAN LLP

Jan R. Adams, M.D.
November 13, 2007
Page 2

In addition, on November 13, 2007, Good Morning America ran a nationally televised news story incorpora ing the alleged quotes that you provided to TMZ (as noted above).

Tl e aforementioned disclosure of private, confidential, and privileged information is in gross violation of California Civil Code Section 56, et seq. and California Evidence Code Section 990, et seq. The disclosure is also a blatant and severe violation of the Health Insurance Portability and Accountability Act (HIPAA), Public Law 104-191, specifically at 45 C.F.R. Part 160 and 164.

Your publicity-seeking foray is nothing short of outrageous, and is in utter disregard of your sworn duties to your patients. Accordingly, demand is hereby made that you, your office, and anyone purporting to act on your behalf, immediately cease and desist any public or private communications concerning Donda West. To the extent that you and your agents continue to publish information about Dr. West or the communications that you had with her, both legal and administrative action will be taken against you and your office.

With respect to your past breach of the Physician/patient privilege, both the Estate and Dr. West's personal representatives hereby reserve any and all rights against you, your agents and your publicist.

Demand is hereby further made that you provide the following to the undersigned in writing, by the close of business on November 14, 2007:

(1) Confirmation that you have ceased and desisted from the dissemination and publication of any further statements about Dr. West or her professional relationship with you;

(2) A list of each and every individual and entity to whom you have disseminated information about Dr. West;

(3) Confirmation that you have contacted each such individual and entity, and specifically instructed each of them to cease and desist from any further dissemination of such information.

Nothing contained herein or omitted herefrom shall be deemed to be a waiver of any of our clients' rights at law or in equity, all such rights being expressly reserved.

Very truly yours,

Brad D. Rose

BDR:mar
cc: Ed McPherson, Esq.
Alison Finley, Esq.

576588

Figure 24 (continued)

It was also inaccurate. I put a call into him to discuss the details of his letter.

"First of all," I said, "No one from our camp [meaning me, my employees, or the employees of Brentwood Surgery Center] had talked to anyone." In fact, the first indication that anyone had even heard anything about it came Monday morning when we received a phone call from a plastic surgeon who had been called by the West family doctor. I informed Mr. Rose that the information about Donda West was not coming from us and was in fact coming from his own camp. I also assured him also that I had hosted a TV show on plastic surgery for five years and, believe me, there was no publicity-seeking behavior on my part.

I did, however, suggest that he should speak to Dr. Aboolian, who apparently, had appeared on an entertainment magazine show and read out loud her medical history from a consultation she had had with him a few months earlier. Mr. Rose at that time informed me that they had associates in the same building as Dr. Aboolian and that he had sent them down the hall to tell that doctor to cease and desist (hmm ...).

At any rate, I followed up our conversation with a letter.

Part of my conversation with Mr. Rose was concerning my ability to respond to inaccuracies in the press. Being a brand attorney, he agreed that I had the right to defend myself and protect my reputation.

That is when Mr. McPherson, who was hired by Rose, joined in the fray. I received a faxed letter at the CNN offices in New York City upon my arrival to Larry King Live. Mr. McPherson threatened that he had filed a complaint with the Medical Board of California demanding that I cancel the interview and that I had been warned not to participate in the interview by the Medical Board, itself. That was not true.

JAN ADAMS MEDICAL GROUP, INC.
11819 Wilshire Blvd., Suite 214
Los Angeles, CA 90025
Telephone (310) 444-8808 Facsimile (310) 444-8809

November 26, 2007

Brad Rose
Pryor Cashman LLP
410 Park Avenue
New York, NY 10022

Dear Mr. Rose:

Per our conversation, I wish to reiterate that neither I nor this office has been disseminating private medical information about any of our patients. I am well aware of California law and HIPAA laws as they apply to this matter.

My first contact with anyone referring to this case or this matter was a plastic surgeon who had called my scrub tech to ask him about the case, purportedly as a result of the West family's private medical doctor calling her. This occurred at 10:00 a.m., Monday morning. At that time, I sat down with my staff and none of them said they had spoken to anyone. So I am going to assume that the information came, though inadvertently, through your camp in their conversation with their private medical doctor for whom I do not have a name. Nonetheless, what is outrageous is your letter suggesting that I somehow was on a "publicity seeking foray." So from my perspective, understand that there has not been a breach of any patient's information, and I would suggest that rather than referring nasty notes to people who you don't know, you solidify your camp so that they stop disseminating information to outside sources.

Should you have any questions, please feel free to contact me at (310) 444-8808.

Sincerely,

Jan R. Adams, M.D.

JRA:ss

Figure 25

11/28/2007 15:26 3102851654 LAW OFFICES PAGE 03

McPherson & Associates

Attorneys at Law

November 20, 2007

VIA TELECOPY NO. (310)284-1654

Thomas Byrne, Esq.
CAREY CARUSO LAW FIRM
425 South Beverly Drive
Beverly Hills, CA 90212

Re: West/Dr. Jan R. Adams
Our File No. 881-1

Dear Mr. Byrne:

This office, along with Brad Rose of Pryor Cashman LLP in New York, represent the family of Dr. Donda C. West. We understand that you are representing Dr. Jan R. Adams in connection with certain medical-related claims. We previously transmitted a letter to Dr. Adams demanding that he cease and desist from his public disclosure of private, confidential, and privileged information about Dr. West and her surgery. Although Dr. Adams has represented to us on several occasions that he has ceased all communication concerning Dr. West, articles and interviews have appeared in *People Magazine* and *The Los Angeles Times*, among other publications, compelling a contrary conclusion.

It is our understanding that Dr. Adams is scheduled to appear on *Larry King Live* tonight, the night of Dr. West's funeral, to discuss, among other things, Dr. West's case, notwithstanding our previous demands.

In order to compel Dr. Adams to refrain from discussing Dr. West or her surgery, and particularly in an effort to compel Dr. Adams not appear on *Larry King Live* tonight, we have filed a Complaint with the Medical Board of California, a copy of which is enclosed for your review. We understand that the Board has contacted Dr. Adams, and has similarly demanded that he cease and desist from any further discussion concerning Dr. West or her case, and has particularly demanded that Dr. Adams not appear on *Larry King Live* tonight to discuss the same.

In that regard, in order to make certain that the family's wishes are made clear, we reiterate our demand that Dr. Adams cease and desist from any further discussion of Dr. West, her surgery, her after care, and anything else relating to her case. More specifically, we demand that Dr. West cancel his appearance on *Larry King Live* tonight, as the subject of Dr. West will most assuredly be discussed on the show.

May 20 08 02:50p 3104448809 p.2

Figure 26

11/20/2007 15:26 3102861554 LAW OFFICES PAGE 04

Thomas Byrne, Esq.
November 20, 2007
Page 2

Nothing contained herein is intended as, nor should be deemed to constitute, a waiver or relinquishment of any of our clients' rights or remedies, whether legal or equitable, all of which are hereby expressly reserved.

Very truly yours,

EDWIN F. McPHERSON, P.C.

EFM/as

cc: Alison Finley, Esq. (via e-mail)
Brad D. Ross, Esq. (via e-mail)

c:\wp\data\[illegible]

Figure 26 (continued)

Retyped copy of letter written by McPherson to Adams November 20, 2007

McPherson & Associate
November 20, 2007

Dear Mr. Byrne:

This office along with Brad Rose of Pryor Cashman LLP in New York, represents the family of Dr. Domda C. West. We understand that you are representing Dr. Jan Adams in connection with certain medical claims. We previously(*illegible word*) a letter to Dr. Adams demanding that he cease and desist from his public disclosure of private confidential, and privileged information about Dr. West and her surgery. Although Dr. Adams has represented to us on several occasions that he ha ceased all communications concerning Dr. West articles and interviews have appeared in People Magazine and *The Los Angeles Times,* among other publications, compelling a contrary conclusion.

It is our understanding that Dr. Adams is scheduled to appear on *Larry King Live* tonight, the night of Dr. West funeral, to discuss among other things Dr. West's case notwithstanding our previous demands.

In order to compel Dr. Adams to refrain from discussing Dr. West or her surgery, and particularly in an effort to compel Dr. Adams not to appear on *Larry King Live* tonight we have filed a Complaint with the Medical Board of California, a copy of which is enclose for your review. We understand that the Board has contacted Dr. Adams and has similarly demanded that he cease and desist from any further discussion concerning Dr. West or her case, and has particularly demanded that Dr. Adams not appear on *Larry King Live* tonight to discuss the case.

In that regard in order to make certain that the family's wishes are made clear, we reiterate our demand that Dr. Adams cease and desist from any further discussion of Dr. West, her surgery, her after care, and anything else relating to her case. More specifically, we demand that Dr. West [sic] cancel his appearance on *Larry King Live* tonight, as the subject of Dr. West will most assuredly be discussed on the show.

Nothing contained herein intended as, nor should be deemed to constitute, a waiver or relinquishment of any of our clients' rights or remedies weather legal or equitable, all of which are hereby expressly reserved.

/s/ Edwin F. McPherson

cc: Alison Finley, Esq.
Brad D. Rose, Esq.

Figure 26 (continued)

I had spoken to no one at the Medical Board and in fact (I learned later) Mr. McPherson had violated the legal profession's code of ethics by threatening action against my license. Besides, the Board has no authority to prevent a physician from conducting an interview. They can question whether the interview violated doctor-patient privilege, but they cannot compel someone not to talk.

I explained to Larry King and his producers that these issues needed to be clarified. I also felt people wouldn't be able to separate me from Donda West so soon after her death. We needed the coroner's report first. In order for people to listen, they first needed to know what happened to her.

Little did I know that the coroner's report would take three months? And so the press was able to spin its stories unchecked. All the while I was requesting of the lawyer's releases to talk about the case. They wouldn't budge.

However, Rose continued to suggest I had a right to defend myself; all the while the attorney he had hired was maneuvering legally to shut me up. (And that is ultimately what came out of it.) I suggested to them that Dr. Aboolian had better have received the same notice. He didn't.

I never really understood at first why they didn't want me talking. I have discussed it with a number of attorneys, and anything I said could ultimately be reviewed by them and used against me in a court of law. Their posture, however, was to generate as much negative press as possible without allowing me an opportunity to respond because of doctor-patient privilege. Regardless of the coroner's determination, they could ruin my reputation anyway.

In a sense, they have succeeded, but certainly not without getting dirty themselves. I personally believe that by helping Scoggins hide his involvement, his negligence in the death of Donda West, both Rose and McPherson have engaged in a conflict of interest and in a sense have harmed the estate of Dr. West, the client they were (supposedly) hired to protect. I believe both of

JAN ADAMS MEDICAL GROUP, INC.
11819 Wilshire Blvd., Suite 214
Los Angeles, CA 90025
Telephone (310) 444-8808 Facsimile (310) 444-8809

November 27, 2007

Edwin F. McPherson, Esq.
McPherson & Associates
1801 Century Park East, 24th Floor
Los Angeles, CA 90067-2326

Dear Mr. McPherson:

I have received your letter dated November 20, 2007. Let me assure you that I have had no conversations concerning your client. I have had discussions with Brad Rose of Pryor Cashman LLP in New York concerning Dr. West and the media and have maintained my agreements with him throughout this ordeal. I find Mr. Rose to be a gentleman and felt that there was no reason whatsoever to doubt his word. I also discussed with him my belief that I have a right to address other issues outside of these circumstances which affect my ability to earn a living, and he agreed.

My conversations with the press have not been about your client, and the slant that reporters take is not something I control. In fact, in one conversation with a reporter I made it perfectly clear that that line of questioning was off limits. She offered that, "Well, what we have to do is test the waters." My point to her was simply that I've made that statement at the beginning and I've made that statement throughout our conversations. I am required by law to honor that and by her asking me questions concerning Dr. West, she is in fact asking me to commit a crime. I would think that the legal scholars would be reviewing that issue on whether or not the press has the right to ask someone who is bound by law to break that law.

In regard to the Medical Board of California, I would hope that you have made the same request concerning Dr. Aboolian in Beverly Hills, California. It is reported that he appeared on television with a patient chart discussing Dr. West's history and physical. If as of 2:30 p.m. PST on November 20, 2007 the Board did not receive the same letter concerning this physician and his "publicity-seeking foray," then I'm going to assume that your attempt to bully me is in fact hypocritical.

Figure 27

Edwin F. McPherson, Esq.
November 27, 2007
Page 2

I certainly look forward to having this entire issue resolved and I certainly respect the wishes of the West family and will continue to honor them. Should you have any questions, please feel free to contact me at (310) 444-8808.

Furthermore, at the request of your office, I have sent a letter and had a conversation detailing the process in obtaining patient records. When we have that information and it is confirmed, you will get a copy of those records.

Very truly yours,

Jan R. Adams, M.D.

JRA:ss

Figure 27 (continued)

these attorneys have willfully and knowingly violated professional codes of conduct, engaged in obstruction of justice, and participated in a criminal conspiracy.

While Mr. Scoggins would like for everyone "to move on" in this matter, I can assure you that the authorities have not. I can assure you that the coroner's office will not take it well that a former cop, who happens to be a nurse, lied to a coroner's investigator. Simply put, that is perjury, and surely, a former cop knows that.

It is only a matter of time before they lodge a formal complaint with the Nursing Board for negligence and perjury; and it is an even shorter matter of time before the LA County prosecutor wants to speak to all of them, including Rose and McPherson.

What I resent most about the behavior of Mr. Scoggins and his attorneys is what their suppression and manipulation of the facts allowed the press to suggest about Dr. West.

Shawn Robinson, from 'Entertainment Tonight', on 'Larry King Live' announced that she had interviewed Donda West a number of times. Then surely **she** knows that Donda West was a smart, confident Black woman who did her homework and made her own decisions. Surely **she** knows Donda West was not some uninformed simpleton taken advantage of by a doctor. Dr. West was the master of her own future.

Even Glenda, her childhood friend, asked me how many times Donda had canceled surgery before deciding to go forward. (Frankly, I'm shocked that Glenda hasn't stood up and screamed to the world, "Wait a minute. This was my best friend and she wasn't stupid." The Donda West I know would have interviewed the doctor and not the other way around.)

I know I still wait for a call that has yet to come. I still wait for a son to say, "I need to hear what happened from you, the doctor. I've had the coroner's report explained to me, but I want to hear it from your mouth."

I know that if it was my mother I'd want to know. And, frankly, I think a son deserves that courtesy.

Incidentally, the L.A. County Coroner's Office is even better than I thought. This is a copy of the complaint they filed with the Nursing Board of the State of California. (I guess that matter of time was shorter than I thought.) After three months of analysis they ruled that "neither anesthesia nor surgery mishaps" were responsible for Donda West's death. After six months and with time to evaluate the lies of her nephew, Mr. Stephan Scoggins, they appear ready to make another determination.

06/17/2008 10:21 FAX 323 224 3678 LA CO CORONER

2007-08227

STATE OF CALIFORNIA
dca
DEPARTMENT OF CONSUMER AFFAIRS

STATE AND CONSUMER SERVICES AGENCY • ARNOLD SCHWARZENEGGER, GOVERNOR

BOARD OF REGISTERED NURSING
P.O. Box 944210, Sacramento, CA 94244-2100
P (916) 322-3350 | www.rn.ca.gov
Ruth Ann Terry, MPH, RN, Executive Officer

COMPLAINT

Please print or type

[illegible]

Name *(Last, First, Middle)*: SCOGGINS, STEPHAN M. RN Number: 458567

Home Address *(Number & Street)*:

City: State: Zip Code:

Employer: SELF EMPLOYED, SEE www.esteemdoctor.com

Business Address *(Number & Street)*:

City: State: Zip Code:

Home Phone: 323-466-2400 Business Phone:

Additional Information *(Birthdate, Former Name, etc.)*:

[illegible]

Name *(Last, First, Middle)*: BERTONE, DENISE CORONER INVESTIGATOR (RN 484547)

Address *(Number & Street)*: LOS ANGELES DEPT. OF CORONER, 1104 NORTH MISSION ROAD

City: LOS ANGELES State: CALIFORNIA Zip Code: 90033

Home Phone: CELL 323-228-8204 Business Phone: 323-343-0714

Relationship to Nurse *(*Patient, Coworker, Friend, etc.)*: CORONER INVESTIGATOR

**If you are the patient or a patient's legal representative, please complete the attached Release Form*

[illegible]

DURING MY INVESTIGATION INTO THE DEATH OF DONDA WEST I WAS CONTACTED BY DR. STEPHAN SCOGGINS. HE WAS INTERVIEWED BY TELEPHONE AND PROVIDED INFORMATION REGARDING THE DEATH OF HIS AUNT. DURING THE INTERVIEW DR. SCOGGINS INDICATED THAT MS. WEST HAD ARRANGED FOR CAREGIVERS TO STAY WITH HER AFTER COSMETIC SURGERY. DR. SCOGGINS INFORMED ME THAT THE CAREGIVERS WERE A FRIEND AND TWO WOMEN WHO HAD BEEN REFERRED BY SURGEON JAN ADAMS M.D. IT WAS LATER LEARNED THAT THE TWO OTHER WOMEN AT THE HOME WERE A FRIEND AND THE DECEDENT'S PERSONAL ASSISTANT, DIANA. DR. SCOGGINS WAS AWARE OF THEIR IDENTITY, YET PROVIDED INCORRECT AND MISLEADING INFORMATION DURING THIS INVESTIGATION. I HAVE BEEN CONTACTED BY DR. ADAMS WHO INFORMED ME THAT HE HAD INTENDED FOR MS. WEST TO GO TO A CENTER WHERE PROFESSIONAL CARE COULD BE PROVIDED AFTER HER SURGERY. I WAS INFORMED BY

Your Signature Date

cpltfrm.doc (rev 12/06, 6/07)

Figure 28

DR. ADAMS THAT HE DISCUSSED THE POST OPERATIVE CARE OF THE DECEDENT WITH DR. SCOGGINS WHO STATED THAT HE WOULD BE ASSUMING CARE OF HIS AUNT. DR. SCOGGINS STATED THAT HE WOULD BE MAKING ARRANGEMENTS FOR MS. WEST TO BE CARED FOR AT HER HOME WHEN IN FACT DR. SCOGGINS DID NOT MAKE ANY SPECIAL ARRANGEMENTS CONCERNING HER CARE. DR. SCOGGINS WAS TO BE THE PRIMARY CARE PROVIDER FOR HIS AUNT AND WAS TO STAY AT HER HOME. ACCORDING TO THE INFORMATION PROVIDED BY DR. SCOGGINS THE MORNING AFTER THE SURGERY HE LEFT THE HOME BECAUSE THE DECEDENT APPEARED TO BE BETTER. MS. WEST WAS LEFT IN THE CARE OF LAY PERSONS. DURING THE INTERVIEW WITH THE DECEDENT'S FRIEND OF 22-YEARS SHE STATED THAT MS. WEST HAD CONTINUED TO EXPERIENCE PAIN AND "HEAVY BREATHING" THROUGHOUT THE AFTERNOON AND EVENING. HER FRIENDS MEDICATED HER WITH VICODIN, BUT IT DID NOT RELIEVE HER DISTRESS. MS. WEST WAS LEFT ALONE AND UNMONITORED WHEN SHE WENT INTO CARDIAC ARREST AT APPROXIMATELY 2000 HOURS ON THE DAY AFTER HER SURGERY. DR. SCOGGINS INDICATED THAT HE HAD LEFT THAT MORNING WITH THE INTENTION TO RETURN LATER AND CARE FOR HIS AUNT. HE DID NOT RETURN TO THE HOME NOR DID HE CALL TO CHECK ON THE DECEDENT. MS. WEST WAS EXPERIENCING SYMPTOMS THAT WOULD HAVE BEEN CONCERNING TO A PRUDENT NURSE. SHE WAS LEFT ALONE DURING THIS TIME. IT IS UNKNOWN WHETHER MEDICAL ATTENTION COULD HAVE SAVED HER LIFE; HOWEVER, DUE TO NEGLECT THIS OPPORTUNITY WAS NEVER PROVIDED. I HAVE BEEN ASKED BY MY SUPERVISORS TO EXPRESS THE CONCERN THAT THIS OFFICE HAS REGARDING THE CARE THAT MS. WEST RECEIVED FOLLOWING HER SURGERY AND TO PROVIDE YOU WITH THE AUTOPSY REPORT AND DOCUMENTATION THAT HAS BEEN RECEIVED FROM DR. ADAMS. ENCLOSED YOU WILL FIND THAT PAPERWORK. PLEASE CONTACT ME WITH ANY ADDITIONAL QUESTIONS OR COMMENTS.

DENISE BERTONE, DEPUTY CORONER
COUNTY OF LOS ANGELES DEPARTMENT OF CORONER
1104 NORTH MISSION ROAD
LOS ANGELES, CA 90033
323-343-0714

cpitfrm.doc (rev 12/06, 0/07)

Figure 28 (continued)

I believe it is time for us to "turn the page". It is time for Mr. Scoggins to step forward and admit the truth about his role in the death of his aunt. It is time for all the opportunists to return to their rocks. It is time for the attorneys involved to stop their misconduct; to stop the obstruction of justice; and to stop the criminal conspiracies. It's time for the press to stop the defamation, and it's time for Donda West's niece to face the truth. Donda West's problem wasn't preop, it was post op. It took place right in her home. Listen to the 911 call.

Those are the facts. At least to the extent that the law would allow me to tell them. I take responsibility for all of it. I recognize that only through accepting it all as my own will I be able to change some of it.

For now I say good bye to a friend. You will always be with me.

APPENDIX

Figure 1: Stephan Scoggins Statement to Coroner's Investigator; Mr. Scoggins, in addition to being an RN, is a former police officer in the state of Oklahoma. He, prior to making his statement, understands that this is a sworn statement and knows that willfully making a false statement to the Coroner's investigator is a crime.

Figure 2: Letter to Dr. Louis Pena, the lead medical examiner in the Donda West case, clarifying false statements made by Mr. Scoggins to the Coroner's investigator.

Figure 3: Confirmation letter from Coroner's office.

Figure 4: Courtesy letter to Brad Rose of Prior Cashman LLP, the litigation attorney for the Estate of Donda West and the surviving personal representatives (i.e. Stephan Scoggins).

Figure 5: Letter from Brad Rose to my attorney Michael Payne; there are two important components of their strategy embedded in his letter: despite allowing Dr. Aboolian to go on TV and speak (they did not file a complaint with the medical board and he has clearly violated the doctor-patient privilege); they go to extreme lengths, including threats, to keep me from talking (they filed a complaint against me and I hadn't said a thing: they are trying to keep me from talking); and, Rose is obviously trying to protect Scoggins even though he knows he committed a crime by lying to the Coroner.

Figure 6: Response from me to Brad Rose concerning his letter to my attorney. (This letter was written out of anger by me and I chose not to forward it to him—there is no reason to be mean—but it does clearly state my feelings. Understand my communication was with the coroner and his investigators-not publishing false and defamatory statements as Mr. Rose would have us believe.)

Figure 7: Confirmation of eligibility to sit for the exam given by the ABPS.

Figure 8: Medical Board of California Accusation. Note false accusation in Paragraph 4, lines 21 and 22. Officer McNurlin testified in court under oath that "at completion of the series of field tests, she did not think the suspect, Dr Adams, was under the influence". Note also the complaint makes no reference to patient care, on the job performance, complaints by colleagues, or referrals by employers.

Figure 9: Medical Board of California: Agreement During Evaluation Process; Self-Referral

Figure 10: Confirmation letter from Bernard Karmatz M.S., LMFT, Diversion Program Case Manager. (NOTE THAT THIS IS DATED OCTOBER 10, 2006.) I first met Mr. Karmatz on December 14, 2006. I soon learned that this was not an oversight on his part. Mr. Karmatz, it turns out, was quite malicious and underhanded. This was to give the impression I had been given two months to comply, not two hours.

Figure 11: Letter from Mr. Karmatz dated January 16, 2007. Mr. Karmatz was trying to exercise control despite the recommendations of his experts.

Figure 12: Response to Mr. Karmatz's letter dated 1/16/07.

Figure 13: More shenanigans on the part of Mr. Karmatz in the name of the Medical Board of California. He suggests that somehow there was some impropriety on my part, but doesn't comment on the facts (i.e. the urine was clear).

Figure 14: Reply to Mr. Karmatz. (Oddly enough I was actually starting to have fun with this.)

Figure 15: Mr. Karmatz changes tactics. He now erroneously tries to suggest that the requests are coming from higher up in the Medical Board's administration. (Problem: I had already had that conversation with his boss before he did.)

Figure 16: Response to Mr. Karmatz's latest attempt at deception. (I told you I was beginning to have fun.)

Figure 17: Mr. Karmatz calls in the cavalry.

Figure 18: Mr. Valine exposed. (Apparently fish do stink from their head.)

Figure 19: Letter from Robin Hollis, Senior investigator the Medical Board of California. (While Ms. Hollis and I did in fact speak on the phone, not one item in her fax was discussed. Conclusion: Another Medical Board manipulation of the facts.)

Figure 20: Response letter to Ms. Hollis. (It's important to understand that the Medical Board represents consumers, not physicians.

Somehow though, they interpret their mandate to mean they don't have to be fair.)

Figure 21: On Larry King Live, Harvey Levin made the claim that 'the Medical Board has been trying to get his license for some time, at least according to its executive director' so I asked them. This was their reply. It seems Harvey misrepresented the truth once again.

Figure 22: Dissolution of Marriage. Item 27 clearly states that "both parties shall be restrained" and not just me as (once again) Harvey implied.

Figure 23: Confirmation letter demonstrating that restraining orders and domestic violence action would be dismissed when Declaration of Disclosures completed. (Apparently lawyers don't want people talking until the checks have cleared in case they get back together or something crazy like that.)

Figure 24: Initial contact letter from Brad Rose of Prior Cashman LLP. Note he does refer to these quotes as alleged and we now know Harvey Levin was less than accurate.

Figure 25: Response to Brad Rose's letter of November 13, 2007.

Figure 26: Initial contact letter from Ed McPherson addressed to attorney Thomas Byrne. Mr. McPherson has overstepped his bounds. Ms Cohen at the Medical Board of California has since informed me that the Medical Board has no such authority. (Our Mr. Mcpherson is a bully.)

Figure 27: Response letter to Mr. McPherson.

Figure 28: Complaint from Denise Bertone, Deputy Coroner, County of Los Angeles, Department of Coroner to the Department of Consumer Affairs, Board of Registered Nursing, State of California: Notice that Mr. Scoggins contacted the Coroner's office and not the other way around. (I suspect this was so that he controlled the flow of information.) The investigator, Ms. Bertone is a nurse herself. Her conclusion on Donda West's death: neglect on the part Mr. Scoggins because of the care Donda West received after surgery.